Dunham Technique
"A Way of Life"

D1479386

Albirda Rose
San Francisco State University

KENDALL/HUNT PUBLISHING COMPANY
2460 Kerper Boulevard P.O. Box 539 Dubuque, Iowa 52004-0539

To the masters who have gone ahead

Pearl Reynolds, John Pratt, and Adrien Ciceron

Contents

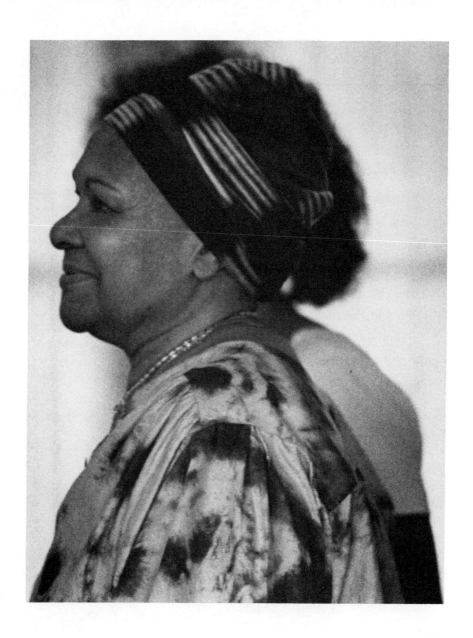

Foreword

It is refreshing and satisfying to read a well prepared textbook on dance technique. For me, it is even more gratifying and encouraging to read a text that deals with Dunham Technique, a technique not easy to describe, as I have found out in efforts to do so for these many years.

When I consider the years of preparation and experience that I have devoted to developing something that can assist in the shaping of people's lives, as well as their bodies, I must say that I am pleased with this work by Dr. Rose.

Dr. Rose is superbly qualified to produce an authoritative work on Dunham Technique. In addition to her duties as a Professor of Dance at San Francisco State University, where she teaches Dunham Technique, Dr. Rose serves as Coordinator of the, "Dunham Technique Seminars," East St. Louis, Ill. She was one of the original organizers of the Seminars, which held its first session in August 1984. The Seminars will have been held for six years as of August 1989.

As an anthropologist and as an educator, it is important to me to have an understanding of, and an appreciation for, people of all races and cultures. As a choreographer, teacher and a performer of dance, I've found wonderful and rewarding ways to express my respect and appreciation for various people and cultures. This is particularly true with reference to the people of the African Diaspora. Dunham Technique is about more than just "dance," or bodily executions. It is about movement, forms, love, hate, death, life, all human emotions. More succinctly, Dunham Technique, which has been called a way of life, is about life in the Universe.

In dealing with these issues in the text, Dr. Rose is careful to remain true to her purpose, which is to present a thorough, but simple work on technique. While she draws upon historical data and takes biographical glimpses into my life, she does so with the intent of showing the relevance of such details in the evolution of Dunham Technique.

If looked upon as a source of technical data on dance, this text will prove to be invaluable. If accepted as a sharing of historical facts, personal knowledge and experience, this work should inspire and motivate.

Dance teachers at all levels, private studios, universities, professional performers, and others, may very well consider this book a collector's item, to be preserved and used for years to come. Students of Dance, as well as Students of Life will find the book to be a manual of instruction on dance and on life. I highly recommend this text to all who have an interest in dance and in people.

Katherine Dunham

Acknowledgments

I wish to extend my sincere appreciation to all who have helped me complete this book:

Thank you, Miss Dunham for the legacy and the opportunity to be a part of it. To my husband, Rev. A. J. Eberhardt who has been patient, loving, caring, and a FANTASTIC Editor. Alicia Pierce, for always listening, reading and holding my hand. Rachel V. Jean-Louis, for your understanding, perception, and courage to make your first drawings. Pamela Hopkinson, for proofreading and asking all the right questions. Jeanelle Stovall for your encouragement and willingness to listen to my dreams. Robert Lee, for caring enough about "Dance" and having faith in me to accomplish the goal. To Dr. Phillip McGee for the initial push. Ellie Louise for your patience and willingness to always work at the last minute. To my Family and Friends who have prayed for me and helped me keep the faith.

Introduction

I was first influenced by Katherine Dunham at the age of seven, when I was a young dance student in a program promoted by the Oakland Parks and Recreation Department. Ruth Beckford, who founded the Dance Division of the Oakland Parks and Recreation Department, was the director of that program at the time. She, like countless others, had been touched by the Dunham mystique, having earlier studied and worked under Dunham in her dance company for a brief period. It was through Ruth Beckford, and by extension through Katherine Dunham, that I was drawn to pursue excellence in dance.

Part of that pursuit towards excellence was to become a Professional Dancer, and a Dance Educator. In 1970, I was one of the last students to take a teachers' course taught by Miss Beckford. This course was privately offered to advanced students who had been chosen by Miss Beckford to be trained to teach Dunham Technique/African-Haitian Dance. In this course we were required to observe a beginning class, participate in the advance class; keep a journal of written description of each exercise taught; and to draw stick figures of such exercise. After observing the beginning class, we were then required to teach each exercise, progressions, and progressions in cultural context. Each lesson that was taught was reviewed and constructive criticism was given by Miss Beckford and the class. Once the course was completed, those of us who had teaching jobs would be observed by Miss Beckford. Each class visited would be reviewed and discussed. This is where I first realized that there was a need for a textbook on Dunham Technique.

As a Professor in Dance of San Francisco State University, where there is a unique undergraduate program in Dance Ethnology, as well as Performance Choreography, Dunham Technique is a strong part of both programs. As I worked in these programs I began to see how a text on Dunham Technique would be helpful in providing a proper understanding of the Technique to teachers and students alike.

To my knowledge, there is no comprehensive, published text on Dunham Technique. Many books, films, and articles have been written that give information about who Katherine Dunham is and what her contributions to the art of dance have been.

Lavinia Williams, one of the original members of The Dunham Company during the period of 1940–1945, furnished material from her personal notes on some aspects of Dunham Technique which was published in "CORD 1980 Dance Research Annual XII." Although extremely important as an historical record, Lavinia Williams' contribution of material on Dunham Technique obviously deals exclusively with an early period lacking in comprehensive detail. This text is designed to fill an apparent void, and to provide a much needed comprehensive detail in easy to understand form.

I am fortunate indeed to have had the privilege of being associated with Ruth Beckford, who represents an important link between Katherine Dunham and myself. Katherine Dunham and Miss Beckford continued to communicate for many years. It is because of the communication between Beckford and Dunham that the legacy of Dunham Technique is being preserved and nurtured in Northern California on a strong and viable level. And the work in Northern California is strong because of the support and approval of Miss Dunham herself.

In 1982, upon the completion of my Doctoral work, I went to East St. Louis, Illinois, to a "Drum and Dance Workshop" in African Dance. While in East St. Louis I became acquainted with Mr. Robert Lee, a long time associate of Miss Dunham. During the two week period of my stay at this workshop, Mr. Lee shared with me much information about the work that Miss Dunham had done as a Professor at Southern Illinois University. He also shared his concern that much of what she had accomplished would not be continued. Memories of these conversations remained with me. I began to look for practical ways through which I could help to preserve the legacy of Katherine Dunham.

In January 1984, I went to Haiti (where Miss Dunham was then in residence) determined to seek her advice and consent regarding the development of seminars and workshops on her technique. Jeanelle Stovall, Executive Director of the Institute for Intercultural Communications, was the key person who paved the way for the events to follow. I was encouraged to learn that Dunham and Stovall had been discussing their concerns for preserving and perpetuating the Dunham Technique, and I was pleased to be a part of the planning that eventually led to the establishment of the Dunham Technique Seminars, the first of which was held in the summer of 1984 in East St. Louis.

These seminars brought together Master Teachers of Dunham Technique and Primitive Rhythms (Traditional Ethnic Dance Forms) teachers, who had been in the original Dunham Company. Participants in the seminars traveled from many countries: Brazil, Columbia, France, Sweden, Senegal, Haiti, Spain, and throughout the United States. Many of these participants were teachers, professors, professional performers, and first time students. The Seminar consisted of exchanging of information, sharing experiences, film watching and listening. My task as coordinator of the seminars was quite broad and varied. The most important task, however, was to document the experiences of learning and sharing within the seminars; engage in dialogue and feedback sessions with Miss Dunham; and to transcribe and synthesize the material which was reviewed into text book structure and form.

Dunham Technique, while it consists of a system of learnable and transferable qualities, its is also dynamic, in that, it continues to incorporate and merge methods of teaching style and application from earlier generations, with the contemporary ideas, methods, and philosophies which emanate from, and are taught by, Katherine Dunham.

For the purpose of this text, I have drawn upon my personal experiences from my first teacher Miss Beckford, from the Master teachers, Miss. Lucille Ellis, Mr. Tommy Gomez, and the late Miss Pearl Reynolds, and of course from my association with Miss Dunham herself.

This text is written with the intent that it may serve as a supplement for both teachers and students. Teachers of Dunham Technique who are familiar with past and present terminology regarding the teaching of certain aspects of the Technique, should have no problem in understanding either the author's style or intent.

It is my hope that this text serves its purpose. It is my humble contribution to the Dunham legacy.

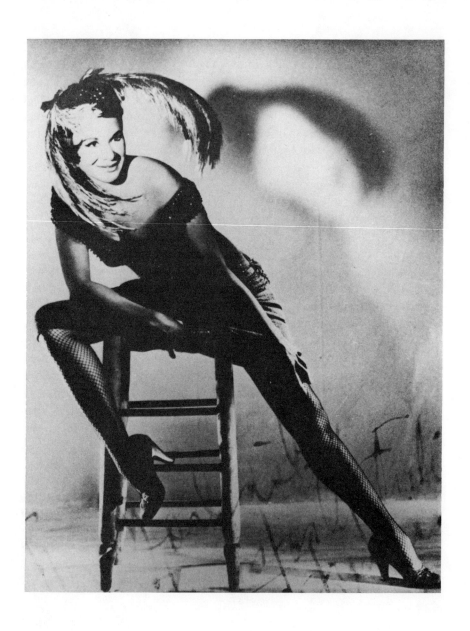

History

Who is Katherine Dunham? Katherine Dunham is a unique and special individual. There are many books and articles that describe who she is and what her accomplishments are. She has been given numerous awards in recognition of her achievements as a writer, anthropologist, choreographer, dancer, and educator. But do any of these give a true and accurate picture of who Katherine Dunham really is? The reader will need to go beyond this text to find the answer.

What we know is, she has contributed to the arts, particularly in Dance, a rich and lasting gift. What she has contributed is the gift of her life. She has given of herself in unmeasurable proportion; what she has given evolves into a way of life that can be shared and duplicated. This way of life is not just in the art of Dance, but in the art of life as well.

The life of Katherine Dunham gives substance and reality to everything that she has contributed, and continues to contribute to "The Art of Dance" and "The Art of Life." The conception of a technique, that is unique to Katherine Dunham, began in Miss Dunham's childhood.

In 1959 Katherine Dunham wrote a book entitled, *"A Touch of Innocence."* In this book Miss Dunham exposes a depth of her essence which, when revealed, gives insight into what Katherine Dunham believes and lives. To Miss Dunham, life is an endless quest to do that which is right and good.

> One spring night as she slept with the window open for the first time since the passing of snow and freezing winter winds and cold Easter rain, the Star woke her with a gentle caress. She opened her eyes in peace, filled with the certainty that she would never again feel the isolation or the fear of loneliness which had haunted her since the days of the closed room upstairs in the Glen Ellyn house. The choreography of her inner being stirred at this instant, Dionysus took possession of her, radiance. Breathlessly she poured into the

night prayer that was to be worded almost identically for the rest of her life.

Help me, star, she said. Help me. Make me strong, give me the courage, make, me know the right thing to do. (Dunham 1959 p156)

Miss Dunham's prayer to "The Star" was for "Help," Strength," and "Courage" to "know the right thing to do." The desire to know the right thing to do has to be the motivating force behind the emerging development of The Dunham Technique.

Far beyond her contributions as dancer, Choreographer, Anthropologist, Educator, Writer, Miss Dunham has contributed generously in the area of humanitarian concerns. Her life has been, and continues to be, one that is devoted to the development of people at all levels, but especially at the lowest levels of society where deprivation and exclusion are very real barriers to creative expression and development. Katherine Dunham is a true Humanist who takes seriously the inherent worth of the individual, no matter what class or culture that individual comes from.

Born in Chicago, Illinois, of a French-Canadian mother and an American father who traced his ancestry as far back as the slave ships from Madagascar, Katherine Dunham is a living legend in the art of dance who, at age 80, continues to give generously from a rich resource of gifts. Dancer, choreographer, actress and writer, as well as educator and anthropologist, she has been called a "multiple personality" because of the multifaceted aspect of her life's work.

Katherine Dunham inherited many of her attributes from her parents. Tall and fair skinned, Fanny June Dunham possessed an outer beauty that seemed to radiate from within. She was a highly intelligent woman of many talents. She was both an educator and a musician. When she was not involved with her duties as an assistant principal at a local school, she enjoyed playing the harp and the organ.

Miss Dunham's father, too, was a man of talents. Albert Dunham, a strong willed, independent business man. For a time he was involved in a profitable but time consuming dry cleaning business. Like Fanny June, Albert Dunham found great pleasure in music. He played the guitar.

Miss Dunham's mother died when Katherine was quite young. Aside from the obvious grief that overwhelms a young child, Fanny June's death brought other complications into the life of young Katherine.

During the next several years of her life, numerous insecurities and uncertainties would be made manifest. Her father, Albert Sr., took the loss of her mother quite hard. His apparent grief ultimately affected Katherine and her brother, Albert Jr., in ways that were confusing to the young children. Soon after the death of their mother, Katherine and Albert Jr. were brought to live with Albert Sr.'s sister, Lula Dunham. Lula worked as a beautician in the already crowded and "bewildering network of the city's black ghetto" (Dunham 1959 p38). Lula's living quarters were a small flat on the southside of Chicago. There was never enough space. Katherine and Albert Jr. had to sleep together in a small bed. Often, dinner consisted of ethnic delicacies bought from the tamale truck that came around each night.

Certain circumstances caused Aunt Lula to give up her beauty shop and to move from her modest flat. Aunt Lula then took Katherine and Albert Jr. with her to live with Lula's sister, Clara Dunham. Clara and her daughter, Irene, had recently moved from Ohio. It was during this period that Katherine was first exposed to the world of music, dance, and theatrical entertainment. She saw and heard about such people as Cole and Johnson, Buck and Bubbles, Bessie Smith, Ida Cox, Ethel Waters, Florence Mills and many others. She witnessed the end of the Minstrel era and the beginning of the Broadway Revue era. Miss Dunham attributed this kind of exposure to her eventual choice of a theatrical career (Dunham 1959 p54).

Katherine demonstrated exceptional talents at an early age. At eleven years of age she finished her last year of Grade school. She wrote a poem that was published in a national magazine. She also wrote a short story about how the turtle got his shell. Katherine also started taking piano lessons at this time.

In high school she was active in dance, basketball and track. Katherine had also participated in minor school productions as a dancer.

Her first performance and choreographic experience occurred when she organized a cabaret for a fund-raising benefit for the local Methodist Church. Included in the planned event was recitation of her original poems, a singing duet with her father, a solo performance of an oriental dance, lead dancer in a chorus of the cakewalk. As a grand finale, Katherine did a performance of the "Russian Princess," a dance she had fallen in love with the previous semester at school.

At eighteen Katherine moved to an apartment her brother had found for her in the city. She took a job as junior librarian in the city. The library "was located in an upper middle-class suburban district of the city where Jews were unwelcome, foreigners of less than two-generation citizenships scarce, and Negroes unknown except as part-

3

time hired help" (Dunham 1959 p309). She received less than favorable reactions from the other employees when she arrived. She realized that it was because she was black.

Katherine benefitted from her job at the library. She developed a love for books. She read almost everything that was available on subjects regarding different people and their cultures.

At the time she was contemplating a college career, Katherine was in a real dilema regarding what courses to take and what major to pursue. Her brother Albert proved to be very instrumental in helping her to select the proper courses that would lead to a degree in anthropology. Katherine entered the University of Chicago with a goal of earning her degree.

Because of her interest in dance, Katherine decided to also take private lessons in dance, as well as enroll in dance courses being offered at the University. The courses included ballet and modern dance. She was influenced by such teachers as Ludmilla Speranzeva and Ruth Page.

In order to pay college expenses, Katherine embarked upon a career as a dance teacher. Her teaching experience began during her first year at the University of Chicago. Her first dance school was opened in Chicago in 1931. The classes were held in a loft and her students were referred to her by friends that she and her brother had made at the University. She taught ballet and modern dance. Through these early experiences she was developing her abilities as a teacher, choreographer and performer simultaneously.

The first effort at establishing a legitimate school of dance was less than a total success for Katherine. The reasons were in no way connected with her skills and commitment, but rather with the inability of the enrollees to pay fees in a timely fashion. She did manage, however, to maintain a few of the original enrollees in her classes. With the assistance of her teacher, Ludmilla Speranzeva, Katherine started a new group. The name was changed to the Negro Dance Group. The name of the group created some strong concerns among the parents of some of the enrollees: "The mothers don't like it. They think the children will be taught Negro dancing-you know, dances like our ancestors back in Africa did" (Biemiller 1969 p84).

Despite some minor setbacks created by the attitudes of some of the parents, Katherine and her group went on to perform in such a successful way that she received more than just attention and acclaim. A woman from the Rosenwald Foundation was in the audience and within the next few days Katherine was offered a fellowship.

4

She received a Julius Rosenwald Traveling Fellowship in 1936 for anthropological research which would take her to the West Indies for one year. In applying for the Fellowship, she was asked what kind of research she had in mind. "She stood up in her tights and first did some movements of the type that were being taught in most schools, 'pretty steps and turns' " (Biemiller 1969 p88). "She then demonstrated in African dance she had choreographed earlier, That's what I'm after. I want to find out why Africans dance, how they started,

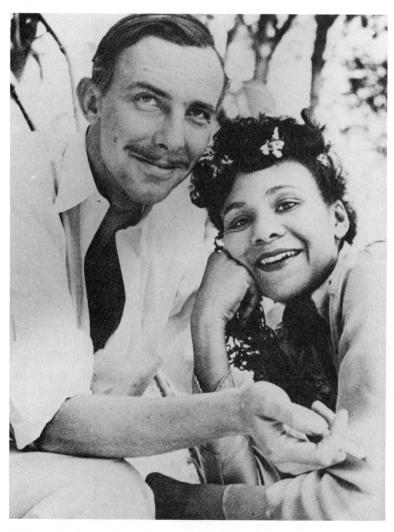

Katherine Dunham and John Pratt married in 1939.

and what this kind of dancing does to people, the life they lead" (Biemiller 1969 p89).

Upon her return from the Rosenwald research project in the West Indies, Miss Dunham was asked to be The director of the Federal Theater in Chicago. It was during this period in her career that Katherine Dunham started a lifetime relationship with Mr. John Pratt, a costume and set designer who later became her husband of forty years. John Pratt died in 1986.

In preparation for her research trip, she enrolled in special courses at Northwestern University. She studied under Dr. Melville Herkovitz, head of the Anthropology Department, Northwestern University. She learned how to work cameras, tape recorders, and motion picture equipment. She learned how to observe with an anthropological eye, as well as how to translate what she observed into report form. What she learned most from Dr. Herskovitz is quoted from Ruth Beckford's biography of Katherine Dunham: "the importance of not offending people in the West Indies and (he) cautioned her to be aware and sensitive to body language and customs" (Beckford 1979 p31). Her trip included Haiti, Jamica, Martinique and Trinidad.

This first travel/research experience in 1936, was more than just a learning experience. The exposure to, and involvement in, the culture of the people of the West Indies taught her much that she would not otherwise have learned. While the learning experience was of tremendous value, Dunham translated the fruits of learning into creative expression.

She wrote many articles and books related to her travel and research. Two such books, *Journey to Accompong* (1946) and *Dances of Haiti* (1950) are reflective of her pilgrimage with people of the West Indies.

Journey To Accompong is a delightful story of a tribe of people living in the isolated mountain regions of Jamaica—the Marrons. *Dances Of Haiti* depicts the culture of the people in all aspects of life—social, sexual, work, religious. Dunham's philosophy of dance would ultimately evolve to a point where she began to perceive dance not simply as physical movement only, but as a way of life:

> Dunham's interest in dance consists of the relationship to all aspects of culture to music, to the plastic and pictoral arts, to religion, recreation, work sexuality and procreation, and social communication. Dance is not just a matter of learning certain "Steps" of physical development, but of learning the meaning of movement, the way of life of a people. (Aschenbrenner 1980 p62)

6

As Dunham developed as a performer, she continued to study and examine cultures and people. As a student of anthropology, she learned how to translate life theories into working methodologies to accomplish her goals as choreographer, teacher, and humanitarian.

The theories that developed as early as her need to understand cultures, were first prompted during her academic training under Dr. Herskovitz. He introduced her to the term "form and function"; Form representing the style and shape of the movement as dance; and Function, representing the need for the dance, what the movement means and what is the significance of the dance (or specific movement) to that cultural system.

While still in college Dunham was not only teaching, she was performing as a dancer as well. She also formed her own company and functioned as choreographer. Under the guidance of Ruth Page, Ludmilla Speranzeva and Mark Tubyfill of the Chicago Opera Company, she became a performer with the Chicago Opera Company.

In 1933 she danced the lead role in Guiablesse, a ballet about the French island of Martinque. This production was choreographed by Ruth Page and produced by the Chicago Civic Opera. She also directed, and appeared in the production of "Run Little Chillun," as Reba. In 1931, working with her own group that had been trained in ballet and modern dance by Mark Turbyfill, the group performed "A Negro Rhapsody." In 1934 she and the group performed at the Chicago World's Fair and at the Lincoln Center for two weeks.

During the early years of her career Miss Dunham's concepts of choreographic style and technique began to crystalize. To Katherine, "the way to plan a dance, was to consider the dancers themselves, choosing steps to fit their particular talents" (Biemiller 1969 p76). In her choreography of "Negro Rhapsody," she spent many hours sketching and planning. She wanted to show that Black people could do more than just soft shoe and the cake walk. The performance was a success.

Miss Dunham's in depth involvement with theater and academic training and research merged to form a synthesis of skill and knowledge. She then had the need to share the information with audiences. Thus, the theory of "Inter Cultural Communication."

Through the process of developing the theory of Intercultural Communication, a unique quality about Dunham's character began to emerge. Her training as a researcher and her drive to perform intersected. At the same time, her need to know about other people, and how their lives are affected by the vicissitudes of life, gave blossom

7

to her humanistic qualities. Her concern with the impoverished people of the world and their cultural enrichness became "Socialization Through the Arts."

It was inevitable that Dunham's research and involvement, even her participation in, and appreciation for, the cultures that she researched would become internalized and become a permanent part of her. The internalized impressions would ultimately become externalized and reflected in artistic, creative expression. The expressions of artistry and creativity were dramatically displayed in many of her earlier works.

In 1938, Dunham created the ballet *L'Ag'Ya* that was inspired from her research in Martinique; this ballet was performed in Chicago at the Federal Theater. Later Dunham went to New York with her newly formed company and performed this ballet at the YMHA. In 1939 Dunham choreographed and directed a show for the International Ladies Garment Worker's Union, *Pins and Needles*. The next show she and her company gave was at the Windsor Theater in New York. The dances were *Tropics and Le Jazz Hot*. It was so successful that they remained for 13 weeks in New York and she was requested to do it in Chicago and then in California. She presented *Rites De Passage* for the first time at a lecture she gave to the faculty at Yale University. Her topic was "A Anthropological Approach to the Theater."

In 1940 and 1941, Dunham and Company performed in a stage production of *Cabin in the Sky*. They later went on tour with it to Los Angeles, and other parts of the United States. While in Los Angeles, Dunham and Company were noticed and received critical acclaim. The professional recognition she and her company received apparently helped to open the way into films.

The first film experience came with the Hollywood production of *Star—Spangled Rhythm,* a war-time entertainment movie. Dunham and Company uniquely hold the distinction of being in the *first* color dance short; it was titled *Carnival Of Rhythm,* which had its story line in Brazil and featured Dunham and Company. They were also cast in the famous film, *Stormy Weather,* which included the who's, who of Blacks in theater at the time: Lena Horne, Cab Calloway, Bill Robinson and many other famous Black stars.

The Dunham Company was on tour in the United States doing an original stage production which she created, *Tropical Revue*. During the tour, she encountered racial injustice and prejudice in several parts of the country. She responded in typical Dunham tenacity and sophis-

8

tication. In a speech made in Kentucky, after a standing ovation and enthusiastic applause from a segregated white audience, she came out on stage and stated "We see by your response you would like us to come back, but we cannot appear where people such as ourselves cannot sit next to people such as you" (Dunham 1984). This is but one example of the many encounters Dunham had throughout the early stages of her career in the United States.

In 1945 Dunham and Company performed on Broadway in *Carib Song* and *Bal Negre,* two of her original choreographic works. In Chicago, she and the Company performed in *Windy City,* in which she did choreography.

Despite her hectic schedule, Dunham also managed to open the Katherine Dunham School Of Cultural Arts, Inc., in 1946 in New York City. Dunham Technique was obviously taught, but classes were also taught in Modern Dance, Tap, Spanish, Oriental, Form and Function, Choreography, Acting, Anthropology and Languages. Part of the staff consisted of many famous teachers, such as Lee Strasberg, Jose Ferrer, Margaret Mead, Jose Limon, Syvilla Fort, Lavinia Williams, and Archie Savage.

Dunham supported her school from monies generated from the performances of her company. The Company went on a world tour from 1947 to 1949. The tour started in Mexico, continued on to Europe, including London, Paris, Antwerp, Brussels, Liege, Nice, Monte Carlo, Italy and Switzerland. Schools were also opened in Paris, Stockholm and Rome, and were staffed by dancers trained by Dunham. The Company was a success wherever it traveled and was received with great enthusiasm. Two of Dunham's most popular pieces of work in Europe were *Shango* and *Woman with a Chigar.*

The tour was broadened to include South America, Europe, North Africa, Canada, Australia, New Zealand, and the Far East. While on tour in Mexico and Rome, Dunham did choreography for movie and television productions in addition to her other stage work. These films show an historical record of Dunham's choreography. In the film *Mambo* of 1954, made in Italy, one scene shows a Company class being taught by Dunham. The Company is shown doing "Fall and Recovery", "Leg Swings" and "Body Rolls."

In 1957, while on tour in Japan, Dunham dissolved the company and remained in Tokyo to write a *Touch of Innocence,* an autobiography about her life as a child. The touring began again in 1960 with travels to Austria, Greece, and Lebanon.

9

In 1961 Dunham returned to her home in Haiti, Habitation Leclerc. Habitation Leclerc was the inspiration for her book, *Island Possessed*. It is her present island residence. Upon her return to the States in 1962, she presented a new dance *Bamboche,* which was based on her work in Haiti. *Bamboche,* included dancers from Africa. Among them were the Royal Dancers of Morocco. In 1963, Dunham was commissioned to do the choreography for the Metropolitan Opera's production of *Aida.*

In 1964, Dunham added a new career. She was name Artist-In-Residence at Southern Illinois University (SIU), in East St. Louis, and consequently did the choreography for a university stage production of *Faust,* and other productions. For a brief period in 1966, Dunham accepted an invitation from the government of Senegal to train the National Ballet of Senegal. She returned to the University in 1967 to continue her work.

East St. Louis, Illinois, became Dunham's second residence. It was here that the Performing Arts Training Center (PATC) was established. Students from the Center performed within the community and throughout the midwest. Although they were not considered a professional company, the students were given good reviews by local arts critics. In 1972, the first performance of Scott Joplin's Folk Opera *Treemonisha* was performed by PATC. The production was performed and filmed at Wolf Trap Farm Park for the Performing Arts in Virginia.

While at SIU, Dunham brought former Company members to help in the teaching and training of the students. The training included Cultural Arts, Drama, Language, and Anthropology.

During Miss Dunham's tenure at SIU, her technique was being refined and defined by her and other master teachers. The recording of each of these classes show a clear chronological development and synthesis of Dunham's Technique. From the beauty of the barre exercise, to the mastering of the progressions, which incorporated integrated rhythmical structures, isolation of body parts, and student comprehension of the exercises and movement.

In 1978, Dunham established the Katherine Dunham Museum in East St. Louis, Illinois, under the aegis of the Dunham Fund for Research and Development of Cultural Arts. The Museum displays many of the Dunham collections from Africa, Haiti, and South America. The collection includes paintings, sculptures, musical instruments, and costumes that Dunham wore throughout her performing career.

In 1979, Dunham received the Albert Schweitzer Award for her contribution to the performing arts and her humanitarian work. On that special evening three generations of Dunham dancers performed. There were students from The Performing Arts Training Center, as well as former Company members. Both students and professionals were brought together again by Miss Dunham in 1980 to do a filmed performance in Dance In America, a series for WNET Public Broadcasting Services.

In 1983, Katherine Dunham was one of five artists to receive the Kennedy Center Honors Award. In 1986 she received the Samuel H. Scripps American Dance Festival Award. She was appointed Distinguished Fellow of the United States Fullbright Commission in celebration of the 40th anniversary of the Commission. She represented the Commission in Brazil. While in Brazil she received tremendous acclaim, including awards, The Legion Of Honor and Merit, and The Gold Medal of the Braizilian Committee on Dance, in affiliation with UNESCO. In 1987 she received the Candance Trailbrazer Award from the National Coalition of 100 Black Women, and was inducted into the National Museum of Dance Hall of Fame in Saratoga Springs, New York.

In December 1987, The Alvin Ailey Company payed tribute to Katherine Dunham in a full evening performance of *The Magic of Katherine Dunham.* Many of the original works of the Dunham Company were included. The work was choreographed, staged and directed by Katherine Dunham.

Katherine Dunham is presently active in her role as Director Of The Institute For Intercultural Communication. She continues to oversee and direct the work of the Dunham Children's Workshop, which is a performing group of children ranging from age 5 to 15. The Dunham Technique Seminars are held every summer in East St. Louis where participants in the seminars travel from many countries: Brazil, Colombia, France, Sweden, Senegal, Haiti and Spain. Participants from with the United States have come from over a dozen states.

CONCLUSION

Katherine Dunham's career can never be divorced from her life. Throughout her career she has had a consistent quest that has characterized her whole life. That quest is a need to know and understand people and their culture.

In pursuit of the quest, she developed a philosophy of life out of which she built three theoretical models. She believes that these models, "Form and Function," "Intercultural Communication," and "Socialization Through The Arts" will enhance the quality of one's life.

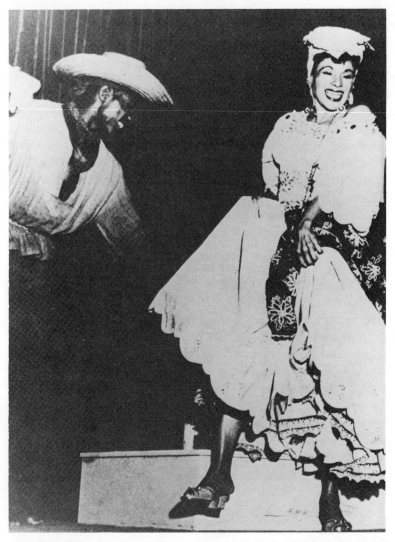

Katherine Dunham and Vanoye Aïken in *Acaraje* at Ciro's in Hollywood in 1955.

The theories became the foundation for the technique that she has refined and defined throughout her life's work: to share, to teach, and to enrich the lives of others. In her work in East St. Louis, Illinois, Dunham continues to pursue her goal of assisting people in their need to know themselves. She uses the art of dance as one means of accomplishing this task.

2

Theories and Methodologies

Dunham Technique is physical and emotional. The Technique presents a mental manifestation of Miss Dunham's years of observing, studying, assimilating, creating, understanding, and living. Dunham Technique uses all the physical elements of dance: space, time, force, quality, isolation, locomotor, and non-locomotor movements. According to Miss Dunham, "Dunham Technique is a series of movement patterns, isolations, progressions and exercises based on primitive rhythms in dance. These patterns create an awareness of time, space, form and function derived from their most basic interrelationship. Dunham Technique is a series of exercises and movement forms, that if mastered, will flow in a logical order into combination of movement and choreographic patterns" (Dunham 1974 p3).

These movement patterns, which emanate from primitive rhythms in dance, provide the student-dancer with the opportunity to recognize and understand human anatomy, its potential and its limitations. "These exercises, their combinations, variations, and choreographic patterns, must be performed with conscious objectives in mind which do not lose sight of the interrelationships between form and function" (Dunham 1974 p5).

For the last 50 years, Dunham Technique has been used to train the professional dancer throughout the world. The Technique has also been used as a tool by both the amateur and professional dancer to facilitate an understanding of culture.

The three theoretical models that Dunham has developed over the past fifty years are used by both teacher and student. These models must be understood in order to execute the technique on the highest level. The three models are:

1. Form and Function
2. Intercultural Communication
3. Socialization Through the Arts

The first model, "Form and Function", is used for understanding dances and specific dance movement. It shows how dance relates to the overall cultural patterns inherent in a particular culture's belief system. For every dance form there is a specific function. For instance, Miss Dunham States in her book. . . .

In the funeral dance the externalization of grief; the social dances, exhibitionism and sexual selection along with social cohesion; in the ceremonial dances, group "ethos" solidarity in an established mechanism of worship, whether through hypnosis, hysteria, or ecstasy. (Dunham 1941 p56)

The second model, "Intercultural Communication," builds on the first. This model, however, is used as a method for gaining a universal understanding and acceptance of others. Dunham believes that through dance and through dance theater, information can be gathered about one's own culture and others. This information assists basic understanding between culture groups, and allows for greater communication, understanding and acceptance of differences:

Dunham uses the theater and all of its techniques in order to be an effective communicator in the medium and culture in which she is operating; without such communication she can be neither anthropologist nor artist, since the conscious mental set of her audience is foreign to the insights she strives to convey. (Aschenbrenner 1981 p56)

These two theoretical models naturally lead into the last, which is "Socialization Through The Arts." This model is used to train people not only as artists, but also as communicators. Dunham believes that if given the opportunity, a student can and will learn important information about him/herself through the art forms of his or her particular culture. Through study and performance of a variety of ethnic art forms, students will gain greater insight about themselves and each other. This will lead to greater clarity in communication as well as better understanding in any setting. This model provides the student with a greater self awareness and thus reflects in the larger social structure in which he/she lives. It gives the student the tools and skills to take part in the community as a productive citizen.

Where Miss Dunham began, she has ended. What she intended to function as a means of shared communication has now developed into a Technique that teaches students about cultural differences as well as cultural heritage. The technique incorporates certain needed skills, and qualities such as discipline, concentration, focus, language, rhythmic assessment, spacial awareness, develops ability to interpret and facili-

16

tates creative expression. These are skills and qualities that are needed not only for performance purposes, but also can be applied in one's life. These skills provide a system for success as performing dancers and but also they enable students to achieve excellence in any given field of endeavor. Thus Dunham Technique translates into a way of life.

In order for teachers of The Dunham Technique to comprehensively impart the Philosophy, they must have experienced it in their own lives as dancers and educators. Even though soulful movement usually comes from a student as inherent knowledge, this knowledge still needs the guidance and fine tuning of a sensitive teacher.

The history of Katherine Dunham's life brings a greater understanding of how The Technique developed. In chapter one, the chronological history of Miss Dunham's life gives the background of the technique development.

In this section the attempt is to point out specific references of that history and how those points have contributed to the development of the three theatrical models that have led to the methodology for teaching The Technique.

As a social scientist, Miss Dunham was trained in participant observation an art of obtaining information about people and their culture. She developed methods that demonstrated how individuals and/or groups share their most personal cultural experiences through their dances. Due to her sensitivity as a humanist, Miss Dunham developed her talent as an excellent teacher. She was able to use her talents and create a methodology that reflected cultural aspects of life through dance. The Dunham performers were able to portray real life experiences of a certain culture because they understood both intellectually and emotionally the content of the culture portrayed. As a choreographer Miss Dunham has been able to pass on the visual and emotional components of her philosophy to an audience via her dancers.

> Dunham Technique must be understood in the light of the philosophy and aesthetic of the larger system from which it derives. (Thompson 1978 p14)

The Technique allows one to understand a culture, or many cultures, through dance. Miss Dunham's quest to understand other cultures began while she studied to be an anthropologist. She found that an understanding of different cultures takes place when one is immersed in the culture. Through experiencing other ways of living, especially through the dances, knowledge is acquired.

The development of The Dunham Technique simultaneously began with her academic studies as an undergraduate student in anthropology at the University of Chicago. Her studies took her to the Caribbean Islands of Jamaica, Martinique, Trinidad and Haiti.

> One of my absorbing interests has been the interrelation of form and function, doubtless sharpened by my Haitian experiences. If the execution of our doings, and the form which this execution takes could be related to a known, conscious function, then we would be far ahead, it seems to me, in the examination and understanding of human behavior and closer to the ability to discriminate in our actions in order to have some quide as to whether or not what we are doing is for the reason that we believe it to be. (Dunham 1969 p129)

Theoretical classification of The Technique appears in the October 1941, article of the *Journal of Education Dance,* "Form and Function of Primitive Dance." Several other articles and books written by Miss Dunham chronicle the continuous development of The Technique. There are also numerous tapes, films and recordings of Miss Dunham actually teaching her technique which reveal valuable information on her nature of the instruction. These tapes span the 15-year period that she worked with the Performance Arts Training Center at Southern Illinois University in the City of East St. Louis. Other professional films show her choreographic work with her company from 1942 through 1965. This material illustrates a continuous and systematic development of The Dunham Technique. The Technique spans over three generations of teachers and influences, as well, three specific periods of movement fusion: "(1) "Fundamental Period" (theme of her technique): (2) "Lyrical period" (smoothes, flows and softens the line of the fundamental); and (3) "Karate A and B Periods" (angular and sharp)" (Beckford 1979 p60).

There is also a fourth period of Dunham Technique. The fourth period began with the start of The Dunham Technique Seminars in 1984. The Seminars brought together Dunham Master teachers in two areas: technique and primitive rhythms, and master drummers, along with old and new students of Dunham technique. These seminars allow for intensive training and blending of the three periods: Fundamental, Lyrical, and Karate, with the added clarification of placement that includes the understanding of energy flow as it relates to the energy centers of the body (Chakras).

The fourth period is the fusion of all the elements of The Technique that return the dance to its natural sources: the inner feeling state of pure balance of body, mind, and soul. The remembrance through muscle, or muscle memory, helps to create and stimulate that energy flow of balance to enhance the physical, spiritual, emotional, and mental towards a greater universal comprehension.

THEORIES

Form and Function

The theory of Form and Function and its importance began to manifest itself through Dunham's choreographic work. Her philosophical foundation and her theoretical approach to her technique start to appear in her earliest writing about her choreographic work, ("L'Ag Ya of Martinique", *Esquire, November, 1939; and "la Boule Blanche", Esquire,* September, 1939). Both of these articles were written about ballets that were a part of her company's earliest repertoire. These dances were based on a particular aspect of life that she found in her research. In the ballet *L'Ag ya* based on the dances of Martinique, Miss Dunham was able to use her unique talent as a choreographer to express the Island peoples' way of life demonstrating their belief system and their history. For example, the description listed in the program of a 1946 performance set the stage for the audience to begin to understand this belief system, and it showed us how Dunham used this method to introduce one culture to another:

> The scene is Vauclin, a tiny 18th century fishing village in Martinique. Loulouse loves and is desired by Alicide, Julot, the villain, repulsed by Loulouse and filled with hatred and desire for revenge, decides to seek the aid of the king of the zombies. Deep in the jungle, Julot fearfully seeks the lair of the zombies and witnesses their strange rites which bring the dead back to life. Frightened, but remembering his purpose, Julot pursues Roi Zombie and obtains the "Cambois," powerful love charm from him. The following evening: It is a time of gaiety, opening with the stately Creole Mazurka or "Mazouk" and moving into the uninhibited excitement of the Beguine. Into this scene enters Julot, horrifying the villagers when he exposes the Covets "Cambois". Even Alcide is under its spell. Now begins the Mjumba, love dance of ancient Africa. As Loulouse falls more and more under the charm, Alcide suddenly defies its powers, breaks loose from the villagers, who protect him, and challenges Julot to the Ag'ya, the fighting dance of Martinique. In L'Ag' ya and its ending is the climax of the forces loosed in magic and superstition. (Clark 1978 p99)

L'Ag Ya is only one example of many ballets in which Miss Dunham depicts a particular way of life and its underlying belief system.

19

This was the first phase of the development and understanding of the importance of form and function. The methodology of form and function, showing how dance relates to a particular cultural pattern and belief system, was used here to introduce people (her audience and dancers) to other cultures. Even in the use of the program notes Dunham was educating her audience through background information which guided the audience further along in its understanding. These developments also set the stage for her theory of "Cultural Communication" through the arts.

Intercultural Communication

Our objective therefore, must be to seek methods for bringing about the essential awareness, through a universal perspective. Only when individuals and nations are able clearly to be aware of theirs and other cultures, see their true values and grasp the universality of these, will the facilities emerge for communication and exchange. (Dunham 1976 p235)

Through the creation of these ballets about the life of a people and their culture, Miss Dunham began to recognize the importance of dance movement and life patterns. The ballets revealed how certain movements related to specific cultural perceptions of life and preparation for certain life events, such as birth, love, or death. Miss Dunham saw clearly how movement has a particular form based on a specific function within a given set of circumstances. Understanding the form and function of these movements and developing it for the stage allow for cultural exchange. Information was being passed on from the choreographer's research to the dancers, from the dancers to the audience.

Dunham Technique is a way of life. For example, when one is learning the way of life of others through their dances, she also learns the meaning of those dances and their specific movements. When the student understands those movements, she will also know their cultural significance. The student thus gains greater insight into a particular belief system. "The System" becomes a way of life as the dancer trains his/her body to become disciplined in understanding movement phrases and rhythmic structures. The dancer allows his/her own being to take on another unfamiliar quality of movement. The individual comes closer to other people, and comes to know oneself through movement patterns and rhythmic structures. These are the goals of "The System." Miss Dunham states:

20

Most of my adult and performing years were spent in creating from Primitive societies a technique and language of dance that would satisfy the demands of western, later world theatre. A holistic approach, taking into account physical structure, personality, culture, the variables within an individual or a society which would make a dynamic, complete, ecstatic experience for performer as well as observer. (Dunham 1986 unpublished)

Dunham expanded these theories which she developed as teaching models, thus paralleling The Technique to the way of life of an unknown culture. It was also a way of life to the dancer. Dunham developed her technique so that it would mold the body in a way that exemplified a particular style. This gave her dancers an authentic look and demonstrated an integrity to the dances they danced. They were simultaneously learning the dances as well as becoming familiar with another culture through language, music, song, and movement. As dancers synchronize with another life style, they inculcate a deeper appreciation of cultural diversity.

Socialization Through the Arts

Dunham Technique must be understood in the light of the philosophy and aesthetics of the larger system from which it derives. Many students have learned Dunham technique without this understanding. The films show the technique explicitly and the system implicitly. The technique is codified, demonstrated, and transmitted daily; The system, on the other hand, is not immediately perceived, not directly demonstrable. Basic Dunham technique involves vigorous work at the bar, isolations, movements, and control of energy flow. The Technique perfects the body; the system clarifies the mind. Such a system decrees change, rigorous self-interrogation. (Thompson 1978 p115)

So, what is this System? Is the "System" truly something that cannot be demonstrated in a technique class? The System can and is demonstrated in technique classes. This "System" is also the element that allows the student to begin to experience "Socialization Through the Arts." Progressions, a combination of movement patterns that allow the student to move across the floor space, defined in a cultural context are but one example.

Another dance of religious ecstasy is the "zepaules," which stresses shoulder action. But to her the ecstasy is of a slightly different quality than in the "yonvalou." It seems that the regular forward-backward jerking of the shoulders, a contraction and expansion of the chest, insures regular breathing, and that this regular breathing brings about hypnotism or auto-intoxication, states border-ing on ecstasy. (Dunham 1941 p3)

Because the elements of dance allow an interplay of the conscious and the unconscious, they are the perfect instruments of the physical form. The human body can embrace all the components of life: emo-tional, mental, physical and spiritual, and bring them together to pro-duce a single creative and artistic expression through dance.

Thompson, also states that the "System clarifies the mind"; And "decrees change, demands rigorous self-interrogation." So what is it about this "System"/Technique that "Clarifies the mind," while de-manding rigorous self-interrogation? The Technique sets up a frame for self-exploration. The dancer has to work toward perfecting the quality of movement within a rhythmic structure, and thereby, is forced to change the rhythmic structure. There are minute details which consistently need development on all levels of human con-sciousness in order to achieve the certain qualities. Therefore, one must understand the **totality** of a particular technique, which means discovering and accepting change. This is "self-interrogation" in terms of values. Dunham Technique fosters the interpretation of val-ues through the elements of dance. It includes the physical, mental, emotional, and spiritual:

> Dunham teaches a respect for truth, an open-mindedness and a pen-chant for self-criticism that is essential for those who would master the technique and learn the system (Thompson 1978 p115)

Self-knowledge is learned through the discipline of The Tech-nique. When the student experiences all of the elements of the tech-nique, i.e. physical, emotional, mental and spiritual; when the student *openly* "lets go" of his/her previous tendency and stylization of movement and incorporates new concepts of movement qualities and rhythmic sensibilities; Then, this growth process repeats itself allow-ing for new levels of self knowledge to emerge. It is this self knowl-edge that allows an individual to sense his place within the society.

Self-knowledge gives insight into the social structure. The student will come to know his/her place in this social structure, and will un-derstand their place and how that relates to the tasks of everyday liv-ing. Self-knowledge also allows for a greater level of self-esteem. Self-interrogation takes place continuously as the student dancer is developing physical and mental discipline, knowledge, and emotional control. Spiritual investigation will give greater insight and under-standing also.

CONCLUSION

Because dance seeks continuously to capture movements of life in a fusion of time, space and motion, the dance is at a given moment the most accurate chronicle of culture pattern. (Dunham 1976 p236)

Incorporated within Dunham Technique is a working knowledge about the historical and cultural development of dance styles. Therefore it becomes necessary for teachers of The Dunham Technique to have knowledge of these developments of dance styles. Teachers should not only have experienced these styles but be able to demonstrate them and to articulate how they work. This is what Thompson was alluding to when he stated, "The system, on the other hand, is not immediately perceived, not directly demonstrable . . . "many students have learned Dunham Technique without this understanding." Teachers of Dunham Technique should know and understand Dunham Technique and all of its elements, so that its uniqueness will not be lost.

After many efforts to arrive at some conclusive decision when thinking of dance, I have decided upon this, that dance is not a technique but a social act and that dance should return to where it first came from, which is the heart and soul of man, and man's social living. (Dunham 1968 p3)

We, as twentieth century artists have always developed the discipline to perfect the physical elements of technique. Miss Dunham accomplished this as seen by the beauty of her company's technical ability. She also captured the beauty and the soul of humankind within the social environment through her choreography. Her choreography reflects life's conflicts, joys, and accomplishments.

The Dunham Technique works to impart the "System" in total. That is technical or mechanical movement that evolves from within the student. Body and soul must join in the expression of emotions that are real to the individual. The emotions have been awakened by an awareness of changing realities of life. A teacher of Dunham Technique must impart the "System" of The Technique to the students as accurately as the physical elements; if not, this would be leaving students with the presence of mechanical movement but the absence of soulful movement.

Philosophy

In the two previous chapters I have sought to reinforce Miss Dunham's idea that Dunham technique is a "Way of Life." This idea is based on Miss Dunham's anthropological studies and the development of three theories which were incorporated into teaching models. Within each of these models the awareness of how the elements of human existence work together in harmony for positive existence as a whole, was formulated through the fusion of the **physical, mental, emotional, and spiritual.** The theory of **form and function** uses the physical; **intercultural communication** and **socialization through the arts** uses mental and emotional; and the implementation of all three models uses the spiritual, which is the inner focus towards self-knowledge.

In 1972 Dunham presented a commencement address at MacMurray College, Jacksonville, Illinois. On this occasion she was presented an Honorary Degree as Doctor of Humane Letters. Her speech was entitled, "Reflections on Survival." In this speech Dunham describes three principles: *Self-Knowledge, Detachment,* and *Discrimination.* She details how she applied these principles in teaching and demonstrating the Technique during her years of growth as a teacher, performer, director and choreographer. The three principles are applied in such a way, so as to show how Dunham utilizes dance as a means of training a student to become totally competent and balanced, not just in dance only, but in other areas of life as well. She realized that without balance there would not be the good dancer.

> Of course it would be good if we could know ourselves through faith and Introspection . . . (Dunham 1972 p16)

SELF-KNOWLEDGE

Dunham uses the principle of Self-Knowledge in a way that leads the student to look within himself. This personal introspection facilitates the merging and synchronization of the physical, emotional, mental and spiritual components of the body needed to develop the dancer. Dunham teaches the principle of Self-Knowledge to assist the dancer in learning the art of personal survival, both, as an artist, and as a child of the universe.

Self-Knowledge, the sum total of faith in oneself to move to feel, to know, and to use for self and others, to give through the motion of the body what we call dance. This is the blending which creates the balanced person on stage, in the classroom, and in one's own private life.

DETACHMENT

Miss Dunham describes the terms "Discrimination" and "Detachment" in the speech of 1972, is a continuation of the development of that balance.

> As a survival measure, *Detachment,* is a dangerous word and must be immediately defined and qualified. Detachment without feeling creates a void of uninvolvement and noncommitment. The Detachment I am speaking of is one of involvement and feeling, and yet of non-possessiveness. It is non-exploitative, capable of objective judgement. (Dunham 1972 p15)

"Involvement, and feeling"—not possessive, non-exploitive: In order to master The Technique a student must bring oneself into the learning environment totally. The feeling state must be attached, open to new emotion in order to totally comprehend movement through one's kinesthetic senses.

"Capable of Objective Judgement"—The responsibility of objectivity lies primarily with the teacher. The teacher must take into consideration the whole, what works and what doesn't and why. These principles are applied within the learning environment, and a positive energy flow is allowed to evolve.

Dunham uses the word Detachment as defined from the French word, "Desinteresse",

> . . . is closer to my interpretation of detachment—that which does not act by material, moral, or personal motives . . . we are able to see dispassionately, but at the same time compassionately. (Dunham 1972 p15)

According to Miss Dunham, the principle of Detachment is taught in order to help the student develop both, as a dancer and as an individual.

DISCRIMINATION

The teacher and student should know when and how to *discriminate* between making necessary and unnecessary choices. Dunham has this to say about discrimination:

> Let us look into the problem of how to choose, select, *discriminate* between good and evil, constructive and destructive, harmony and dis-harmony, both in our individual and social lives, and how to select with wisdom alternative acts set before us. . . . To make clear distinctions between or amongst the essential and the superfluous. (Dunham 1972 p15)

Synchronization of body rhythms creates harmony. Dis-harmony causes destructiveness. To dance in harmony with one's self, or in harmony with others, brings about a joy that can be felt by both the professional and non-professional dancer. The superficial attachment of movement for style only is not necessarily good dance. Understanding the essentials of quality movement, which merge all of the components of being human, is the sign of the wise and good dancer.

Each aspect of The Technique is described for practical application. The descriptions are simple and are explained in basic dance language. As The Technique is being taught, the teacher and the student should take into consideration the learning environment, the objectives of the class, and the individual attitudes of each student. Essentials for achieving good results are positive attitude, favorable environment, and a realistic expectation that is based upon an awareness of one's level of commitment.

The positive energy that is brought into the learning environment by each individual teacher and student, where the main focus is on body motion that is being prompted by vibrating drums, creates a corporate energy that engulfs the whole group. Negative drum vibrations could emanate from negative energy being transmitted by drummers, teacher, or students, and could negate the flow of positive energy from all. All things must be in harmony—drummers, movement introduced by the teacher, students who are willing to submit to the drum vibration and the movements or rhythms presented.

The **Physical** mechanics of the body in connection with a **Mental** state of conscious effort, will create a feeling state, thus allowing the **Emotions** to respond to one's personal **Spirituality.** To know oneself, or to be aware of self, brings about self knowledge. This inner focus tends to create an awareness of what one's contribution is to the whole. The wise teacher and student will ask: Who am I? Why am I here? What do I want from this experience? Personal introspection tends to produce the potential for greater personal development. Miss Dunham states:

> Coupled with this spiritual revelation is the physical, facilitated in its responses by a body well muscled and in classic balance. The Body is a built-in part, a necessary part of the full realization of our own rhythmic pattern. There is a great sense of arriving, of invincibility, when flesh and spirit are together in this truth. Every movement of the body is in harmony with spirit. There is an eternal choreographic pattern sometimes taking external form, sometimes remaining within, but always there. This is what dance has meant to me, and every day, each split moment of every day I dance. (Dunham 1972 p13)

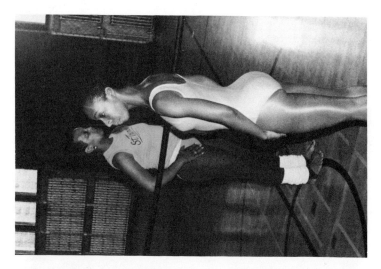

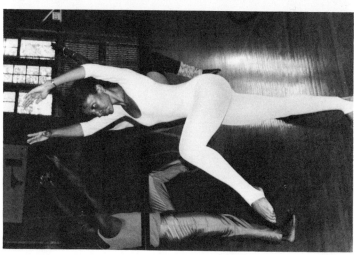

Photos by poet Eugene B. Redmond.

Practical Application

So far I have discussed the Historical background, The Theories, and the Philosophy from which Dunham Technique has evolved. It is clear to me that in terms of who she is and what she believes in, Katherine Dunham is both the spring and the fountain of Dunham Technique. Her life as a person, student, teacher, researcher, artist, and choreographer, has produced a technique that is both learnable and transferrable. It is the learnable and transferrable aspects of The Technique that are the subject of this chapter.

For both student and teacher, an adherence to certain basics in the practical application of The Technique is expected in order to achieve desired objectives.

The purpose in this chapter is to present in sequence, a description of the exercises and movements, which are characteristic of a Dunham Technique class.

BREATHING

Breathing

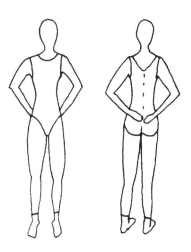

At the start of any class, one usually comes with an intent and complete focus as to what their individual objective is for that day. When Miss Dunham starts a class, the first physical preparation is to begin with Breathing, which is a basic part of The Technique.

Breathing is basic to life. It is a life force. Dunham used the breathing exercise to cleanse the body. Learning how to breathe appropriately within one's own rhythmic

31

force allows the student to prepare the body for strenuous activity and focus the mind towards conscious disciplined activity.

The student faces the front of the studio with feet parallel, arms folded to the back. The hands are closed and resting on the lower back. The eye focus is straight ahead. The breath is taken in through the nostrils filling the lower abdominal cavity. The ribs and shoulders should not rise. As the air is released through the mouth a throaty sound should accompany it. This exercise is repeated rhythmically at the discretion of the teacher.

BARRE WORK

Sequence 1   Placement

The student faces the barre, feet parallel and as wide apart as his/her shoulders, arms are down to the side, focusing straight ahead. The arms are placed at the insertion of the hip joints, palms flat, fingers facing in.

Sequence 2   Dunham Presentation

This is the Dunham presentation of the arms. On the count that is set, the student begins to raise the arms forward, in four counts. Half-

Pushing-In

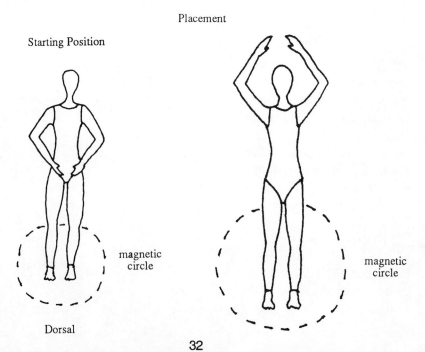

Placement

Starting Position

magnetic circle

magnetic circle

Dorsal

32

way up, the arms stop, palms are flat, elbows and shoulders are balanced equally. In this halfway position hold for four counts. The arms continue raising above the head (hands slightly in front of face) and are held in this position for four counts

While holding the position above, the student checks for correct body alignment:

- The head is centered
- The shoulders are well balanced over the chest area
- The chest lined up over the waistline
- Waistline is directly over hips through to the thighs
- Thighs directly over the knee
- The knees directly over the toes
- Feet in parallel (approximately 8 inches apart)

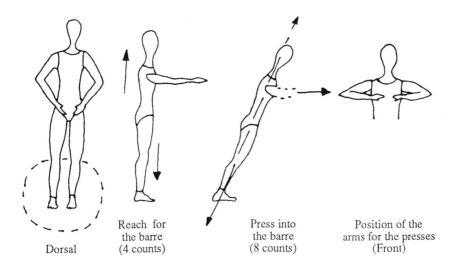

| Dorsal | Reach for the barre (4 counts) | Press into the barre (8 counts) | Position of the arms for the presses (Front) |

Sequence 3 Plie, Releve

From *Sequence 2,* the arms lower (in four counts) from above the head. The focus of the student is directed towards their own body, thus being aware of where they are in space, and not being concerned with what is around them. The student should develop an inner focus so as to avoid unnecessary distractions. The focus should be on the drums (or accompaniment) and the instructor's voice.

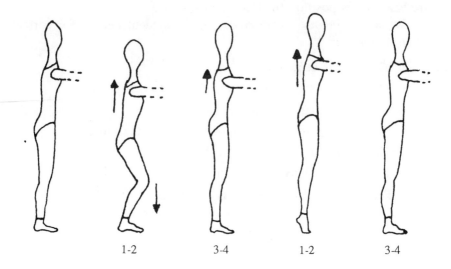

1-2   3-4   1-2   3-4

The Dunham presentation continues. Depending upon the instructor, it may be repeated for two sets of four or two sets of eight, or four sets of four, counting:

- Count 1,2 Arms lifted and forward to halfway
         3,4 Hold
- Count 1,2 Continue lifting above the head
         3,4 Hold
- Count 1,2 Arms lower to halfway
         3,4 Hold
- Count 1,2 Continue lowering the arm
         3,4 Hold, back to the barre

With the hands placed on the barr, the student begins to do plies. Again this is a time when the student should check their alignment and their focus.

- Slowly counting
- Count 1,2 Demi-plie in parallel
         3,4 Raise up, straightening legs,
- Repeat 4 times.

34

- Then, starting from straight leg position,
- Count 1,2 Releve
          3,4 Come down, into plie to straight leg, flat foot
- Then reverse,
- Count 1,2 Plie
          3,4 Up, to straightened position
- Count 1,2 Releve, holding balance
          3,4 Hold

While holding one's balance, the hands should be lifted from the barre into the Dunham presentation of the arms above the head. The arms lift up in four counts. When the arms are above the head in the holding position, the instructor should check for correct body alignment. The shoulders are not raised but are completely balanced with the arms circling above the head so that you have a nice presentation where the face and the chin are lifted, the buttocks are tucked under, the abdominal muscles are working held in, long and lifted.

Next, the student will lower from releve to flat foot and return the arms in four counts to the starting position to complete this sequence; after making necessary adjustments the pushing-in sequence would begin.

Sequence 4 Pelvic Placement

Pelvic placement teaches students to understand their body alignment and where they are exactly in space. Students begin at the barre with the feet in first position (parallel), hands slightly on the barre. Students can begin to do plies, straighten the legs, releves:

- Count 1,2 Plie
          1,2 Slowly straighten
          1,2 Releve
          1,2 Straighten
          1,2 Plie
          1,2 Straighten
          1,2 Releve

This should be repeated as many times as the instructor feels is necessary. Finally, holding in plie, isolation of the pelvis begins.

The pelvis should contract forward, return to center (check for alignment: head between shoulders, shoulders over chest, chest over the waistline, abdomen pulled in, long tailbone-center position), hips isolate to the back (hyper-extended placement), return to center. Only the pelvis moves. Repeat this at a slow tempo until understood by the students, then movement can be done at a quicker tempo:

- Count 1 & Forward pelvis
         2 & Center pelvis
         3 & Back pelvis
         4   Center pelvis

Pelvic Placement

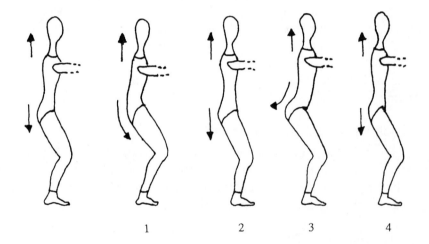

| | 1 | 2 | 3 | 4 |

- or At the quicker tempo,
- Count 1   Forward pelvis
         2   Center pelvis
         3   Back pelvis
         4   Center pelvis

Hold for 4 counts, pelvis contracted in the forward position, let go of the barr, arms falling down to the sides, place upper torso over hips, heels come up slightly, knees bent as student goes into a deeper hinged position with the pelvis forward.

Once again the student has the opportunity to begin to understand what is meant by pelvic placement. The body should return to correct alignment by placing the heels of the foot back on the floor. The pelvis returns to the center position and the upper torso follows, the knees straighten.

Sequence 5 Pushing-In

Again, the heels are as wide apart as the shoulders in the parallel position; the hands are placed on the barre lightly; the body is one total complete entity; (not breaking at the waist or hip) the student begins to push-in towards the barre in that complete entity.

In 8 counts arms bend at the elbow, as the weight goes into the barre, the palms are flat against the barre, fingers facing each other, (by having the hand and fingers in this position the student continues to maintain the force field of energy that he/she has developed in *Sequence 1*.

Sequence 6 Flat Back

In the flat back position, the body bends at the torso, the arms are opened wider, hands placed on the barre, the neck is extended long, towards the barre, the legs are straight, the heels stay flat on the floor. The students will move into this position in an 8-count sequence once he/she has accomplished the pushing-in sequence.

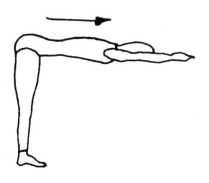

Twice in 8 counts
Twice in 4 counts
Four times in 2 counts
Eight times in 1 count

Press into flat back
(8 counts)

Flattening the back (counting 1-2-3-4), the upper body never comes up all the way to standing height, the emphasis is to slightly push the back into a flat back position and at the same time pull-in with the abdominal muscles for lower back support, opening the sternum, opening the upper back wider, the arms and the head stay in alignment. The abdominal muscles are still working so that the students begin to feel elongated, although bent at the hip joint, feeling that their head and spine are continuously stretching forward, over the toes. The body is well balanced and controlled.

This sequence should be repeated twice to the count of 8, twice to the count of 4, twice in 2's, then in four sets of 1's with the legs straight.

At the completion of the four sets of 1's, the students hold the flat back (SEQUENCE 6), then go on to body rolls.

Sequence 7 Body Rolls

Through the development of strength and abdominal muscle control from the previous exercise, the student should have a visual working knowledge of the pelvic area.

At this point the student begins to understand the use of the pelvic area. The large gluteus maximus muscles are used in this position where the pelvis inserts into the thigh muscles and the front area of the pelvic girdle. In the flat back position, the student will contract and release the pelvic area from both the front and back (this may take some work). The instructor should have the students place their fingers into the soft tissue area in order for them to feel where the start of the movement should begin.

The fingers should be placed so that they can feel the contraction and release of the muscles. This could be a very difficult aspect of the technique, but once perfected the rest will flow accordingly. The instructor must make the students aware of where the pelvic girdle and where the pelvic contraction exists. The instructor should note that this entire sequence is done in the flat back position and that the "release" does not indicate hyper extension of the pelvis or lower back, but that the back returns always to the flat back position.

- In the pelvic area
  contract and release
  should be repeated approximately four
  times working each specific area

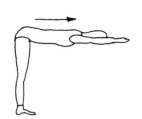 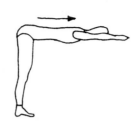

Pelvis contraction
(2 counts)

Stretch into a flat back
starting with the head
(2 counts)

(REPEAT)

Pelvis
first

Head
first

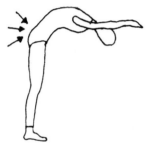 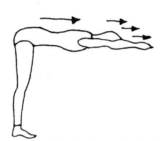

Full contraction
starting with the pelvis
(4 counts)

Stretch into a flat back
starting with the head
(4 counts)

(REPEAT)

- Using the gluteus
  contract and release,
  and repeat 4 times
- Move into the lower back area
  contract and release 4 times
  (The student is still in the flat back position)
- Move up into the middle back area

contract and release four times
- Upper back area

contract and release,

repeat four times
- Head area
- Then all of these body parts are put together in continuous motion to complete the body roll.

The completion of the body rolls is in 4 slow counts, repeated in at least four sets:
- Count 1 Pelvic and gluteus areas
-        2 Lower back
-        3 Middle back
-        4 Upper back connected to the head, the neck into the top of the head reaching forward over the toes so that the body feels as though it will fall forward into the wall.

This should be repeated slowly, approximately four to eight times in measures of four; thus you have:
- Count 1,2,3,4   Reach
- Count 1,2,3,   Contract
-        4   Reach
- Count 1,2   Contract
-        3,4   Release, making a nice elongated body

At the completion of the body rolls in flat back, the students should hold for 4 counts, again focusing and finding their balance,

Body Rolls (ending)

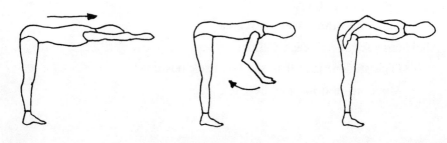

being in total alignment; then the right hand comes off the barre, sweeps down along the right side of the hip, elbow comes up, palm reaching down with slightly cupped hand; then repeat with the left hand.

Depending of the level of the student, this could be done with both arms together or one arm at two different counts. Beginners should do one arm off at two different counts so that they can feel where their balance point is, then the other arm comes off in the second count. More advanced students can take off both arms in one count and hold the position, and know where they are in space without losing balance. At the completion of the sets, the flat back position is held.

Then the arms and hands are brought in towards the body, palms facing towards the body, the back is still flat, then starting at the pelvis, the pelvic contraction starts a body roll placing each vertebrae on top of each other, slowly; the pelvis, gluteus, lower back, middle back, upper back, shoulders, neck and head until standing position is reached with proper alignment.

As this is being done, the arms are in a continuous flow of motion. They come up, in 4 counts, above the head. Again the shoulders are down, focus is straight ahead, chin is up and you frame the face as a perfect picture and the entire position is held.

If this is a level 1 class (beginners), this exercise should be done with flat feet; if level 2 or 3 students, they can begin, as they contract, to start the pelvis movements and roll up on 4 or 8 counts. Depending on what the instructor feels is appropriate, they should begin to releve lifting the heels slowly, the arch of the foot, the ball of the foot onto the toes, and hold this position 4 to 8 counts. Again, the student should be aware of their own center, knowing that their pelvis is in alignment, tailbone is long, neck is long, chin is slightly lifted while looking straight ahead, shoulders down and relaxed. Hold, then slowly come down completing the movement in 4 or 8 counts. Arms come back down to the beginning position.

Sequence 8 Fall and Recovery

Start from a parallel base with the feet as wide apart as your shoulders; arms are down to the side. As the arms come up, the back will reach over into the flat back position (as done previously) in 4 or 8, when the position of the flat back is reached. The arms are wide, hands placed on the barre, and the neck is long.

Fall and Recovery - Flat
Starting Position

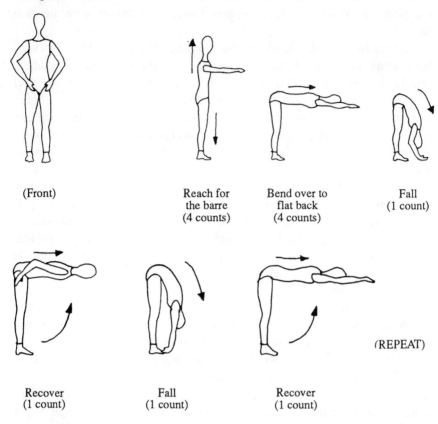

(Front)	Reach for the barre (4 counts)	Bend over to flat back (4 counts)	Fall (1 count)

Recover (1 count)	Fall (1 count)	Recover (1 count)	(REPEAT)

The upper torso and arms drop (as indicated in the exercise explanation—fall and recover), letting the energy fall from the upper body (yet controlled). Because of the generation development of the sequence, the fall has been taught with the head leading the chest. The arms fall to the sides of the legs as the movement occurs.

In the recovery, the impulse from the drop carries the student up toward a rounded back, like a breath phrase, then moves back to a flat back on the recovery. The arms drop down to the sides, in a reverse of the last movement. In recovery the arms are on the side of the body away from the barre.

Then they reverse the motion: the arms go back down along the legs, reach up to the barre and hold, as the flat back is held in the recovery position. So at the completion of the movement, in flat back position, the arms are nice and wide, the back is long and the body weight feels like it is going forward, the top of the head is elongated

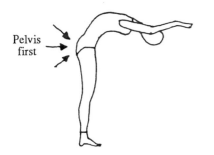

Pelvis
first

Roll: starting with
the pelvis
(2 counts)

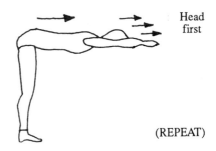

Head
first

(REPEAT)

Release into a flat back:
starting with the head
(2 counts)

and one should feel like he/she is going forward into the barre or wall.

The description of this exercise can be repeated variably for clarity and rhythm; fall and recover, and fall and recover. Exactly how it is said in a vocal rhythm pattern is how it can be done physically.

The student should not 'hit' or cause a strong percussive jolt in the lower back in the recovery. The chest should not push out towards the floor in hyper extension. The movement is a very subtle full drop and then recovery on the breath phase, and a reaching out long with the upper torse as if continuing the body roll. This should be repeated four times. Four falls and recovers are considered 1 set.

If this is a beginning class, this particular exercise with straight legs should continue for the first three to four weeks without any variation until the student truly understands body alignment. If it is a level 2 or 3 class, they can begin falls with straight legs, then add a variation of plie and releve.

Every time the student falls, both knees bend equally and the back is flat—you have a bent position with the back flat, pelvis is lifted, head is long, there is no break at the neck. Hold this position.

- Plie (fall)
- Straighten the legs on recover
- Plie, straighten the legs
- Plie, straighten the legs

Or;
- Fall, plie and
- Fall, straighten the legs

43

Fall and Recovery with Plié

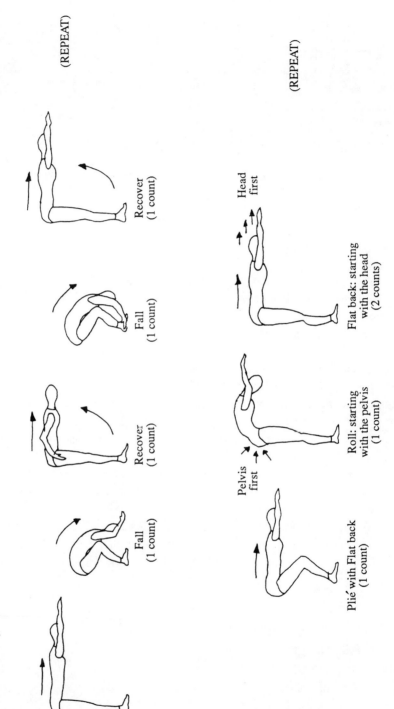

Recover
(1 count)

(REPEAT)

Fall
(1 count)

Recover
(1 count)

Fall
(1 count)

Head
first

Flat back: starting
with the head
(2 counts)

Roll: starting
with the pelvis
(1 count)

Pelvis
first

Plié with Flat back
(1 count)

(REPEAT)

44

And it reverses:

- Fall, plie
- Come up; straighten the legs

Then you reverse the arms as you did before.

Variation 1

This can also be done by intermediate and advanced students from plie to releve and elevation

- Fall, plie
- Straighten up to releve;
- Fall, plie
- Straighten up to releve.

Again the arms stay the same:

- Fall down by the side of the legs, both arms at the same time
- Slight curve in the back, breath phrase
- Reach out on the recovery
- Arms are straight
- Palms down, elbows slightly bent

Variation 2

Once the movement is understood by beginners and has been reviewed for two to three weeks with the straight legs, then a body roll can be added in between two sets (in 4 counts). This is the same body roll done in the beginning of the class in the warm-up area.

- Fall and recover, fall and recover (1 set)
- Fall and recover, fall and recover (2 sets)
- Hold on to the barre
- Contract pelvis: roll pelvis, lower back, middle back, upper back, through neck and head weight is forward (as if one is falling forward)
- Hold (4 counts)
- Hold (4 counts)

Count as follows:

- Count 1   Fall and recover (with the reverse to complete the set)
- 2   Fall and recover

> 3   Fall and recover
>
> 4   Fall and recover

- Hands on the barre holding in the flat back position,
- Count 1   Pelvis

> 2,3   Body roll
>
> 4   Hold

Repeat this sequence as many times as you feel necessary. I strongly suggest that you do this exercise with straight legs in two

Fall and Recovery with Plié and Relevé

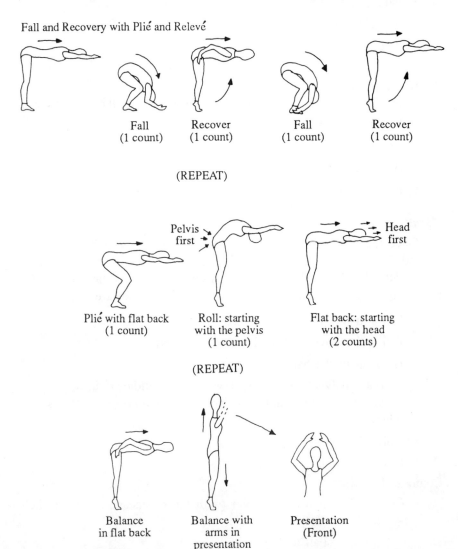

Fall
(1 count)

Recover
(1 count)

Fall
(1 count)

Recover
(1 count)

(REPEAT)

Pelvis
first

Head
first

Plié with flat back
(1 count)

Roll: starting
with the pelvis
(1 count)

Flat back: starting
with the head
(2 counts)

(REPEAT)

Balance
in flat back

Balance with
arms in
presentation

Presentation
(Front)

sets: two sets in plie and two sets in releve. Another variation on the fall and recovery with the body roll (or without depends on the level of the class) is done with a jump:

- Plie, releve, jump
- Plie, releve, jump

The heels leave the floor doing this same sequence with a jump. This can also be done moving across the floor.

Sequence 9 Heel Press

Heel Press is also started with feet in first position (parallel), hands placed lightly on the barre. The right foot is going to go to the side and behind the other foot in the parallel position with the ball of the foot on the floor and the heel of the foot lifted. This exercise stretches the achilles tendon, hamstring, and calf. Here again, the students should be aware of their body alignment.

The starting position is with the heel up, the front leg is straight, and a concentrated effort of correct hip alignment. When the back heel goes down (on the count of 1), the heel of the left foot is on the

Heel Press

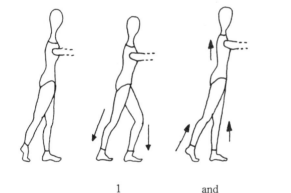

1   and   2...   6 and

47

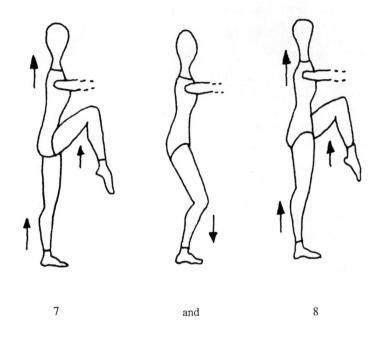

7   and   8

floor and the knee bends. (One leg is straight with the heel down, one leg bent).

The heel then comes up off of the floor and the front leg straightens.

- Count 1   Back heel goes down

  and

  2   Straighten

  and

  3   Up

  and

  4   Straighten

During this time the body is held in a standing position as much as possible, the body alignment has not changed, and there is no rocking in the hips from side to side. If there is a tendency for the student to rock at the hip joints or to allow heels to turn out, turn the heels slightly in a turnout position. You must always correct the position so that the feet stay in parallel and the body alignment stays correct. The wall should seem as if it is going up and down and not in and out.

The heel press can be done with variation on the counts and with the transition taken on each new count. You can have the heel press done in 8 counts with the transition in 7.

- Count 1   Heel down and up through the count

        6   Straighten, and on

        7   Heel down, bring same
leg (right) up
with knee bent, thigh
goes up to chest

        8   Leg goes down, plie
(both knees and heels together at the same time),
opposite leg (left) comes up, goes to the back and
its there on the count of 1 ready to start from the beginning, repeating the exercise on the left side.

This sequence is usually repeated twice with the transition on 7; then twice with the transition on 3; then the transition is on every count. So the transition continues for approximately 8 counts.

Variation 1

Heel press variation in releve with the counts as suggested previously, begin in the same way as above with the right heel back, both heels up. Start in a releve with hands lightly on the barre, head in place, shoulders aligned, pelvis pulled under, long tailbone, abdomen pulled in, and chin lifted. Both heels go down at the same time, front knee bends. The only change is when you go up on releve, both heels are up at the same time and when you go down, the back heel still stretches back and the front heel goes down and the knee bends. You must check that the back heel is not left up in releve when the front knee is bent. The heel must go down in the plie as the back heel goes down, in transition.

Variation 2

Another variation is to do this movement with one hand on the barre standing to the side of the barre so that a new facing is established.

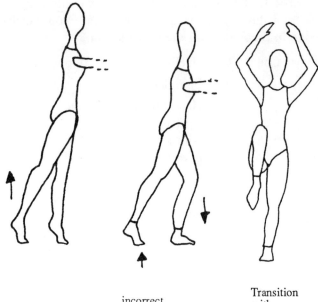

incorrect

Transition
with arms

Variation 3

This can be done with the Dunham presentation of the arms, so that on the transition the arms can go above the head or center depending on the level of the students.

Level 1 students may not always be ready to do releve until a certain amount of time (possibly four to six weeks) and practice has been achieved. The students must completely understand the heel press and the heel press variations before they can go on to a more intense level using the variation of releve.

This particular exercise is very important for body placement and alignment. If the student has understood the earlier pelvis placement and other variations of drop and recovery, then this exercise should be easier.

Again, the instructor should look at the student's total body alignment from the back side. Here you can see whether or not the student understands the parallel position in an open 4th or a parallel position in a 2nd position. The back is straight, the chin is lifted, the chest is lifted, the abdominal muscles pulled up and in.

Sequence 10 Back to the Barre Foot Isolation

Feet in parallel position. Arms relaxed and stretched out and hands placed lightly on the barre. There is no obvious bend in the arms at the elbows. Again, in this position everything is in alignment.

The movement begins with the right foot being extended forward reaching as far as it can go. The foot is pointed and flexed to warm-up the ankle area. There are several variations that can be done depending on the needs of the class. The isolation is the important factor. Pointing and flexing of the foot is repeated. As you point, you reach out and away from your body as far as you can without throwing the body out of alignment. In flex you bring the foot back underneath you so that you are standing again in correct alignment.

- Count 1   Point
-       2   Flex
-       3   Point
-       4   Flex, bring the heel back again.
- Repeat this up to 8 counts on both sides.

Variation 1 Circles

The right foot begins to circle at the ankle, out and away in 8 counts. Again the foot is directly in front of the body (the whole leg) as far as it can go without throwing the body out of alignment. Circle four times to the right, with toes reaching out away from the body; then four times to the left, with toes reaching in towards the body. Four counts right, then four counts left. Repeat with the left side, with the same counts. Always bring the foot back into first position parallel for placement and correction.

Variation 2 Brushes

Another variation is brushes on the floor. The foot is brought out away from the body. Begin by pointing through the toe ball, arch, and heel of the foot, then brush the foot back towards the body (the momentum is through the leg) leading with the heel and repeat the movement. Again depending on the skill level of the class this can be done with straight or plie legs. This is repeated four times right side, then switch to left side. This can be done in parallel and turn-out. An

Heel Press Variation

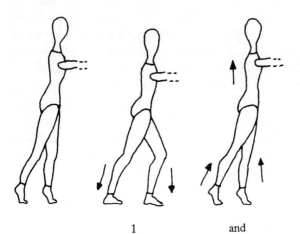

1   and   2...   6 and

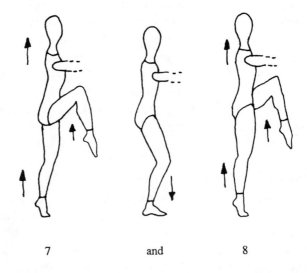

7   and   8

Feet Isolation

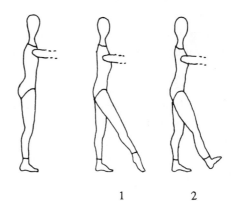

1   2

Feet Isolation Variation

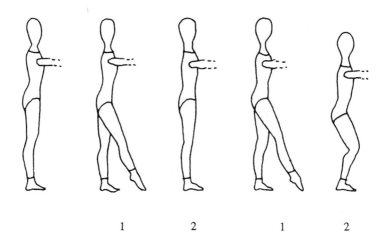

1   2   1   2

added variation to this would include plies after the brushes have been completed, in the same position.

Variation 3 Plie, releve

Repeating the variation above four times, hold, go to releve, hold. Come down in a grand plie slowly then go slowly to straight legs and then go to turnout and repeat the exercise in the new position.

Variation 4 Point, flex

Another variation is repeating the first point-flex sequence, having the foot bring the leg upward as high as it can go without changing the alignment. Starting with the right leg: point, flex, point, flex—bring the whole leg up higher until it is at waist height.

- Count 1 Point
  - 2 Flex
  - 3 Point
  - 4 Flex
  - 5–8 Bring the leg up higher
- Count 1 Point
  - 2 Flex
  - 3 Point
  - 4 Flex
  - 5–8 Bring the leg back down underneath you, repeat on the left leg from beginning point-flex move ment.

Variation 5 Quiver

Bring the leg up with pointed toes, then hold that point as tight as you can. The muscles begin to quiver; your entire muscle and leg joint moves so that it begins to shake or vibrate quickly for 8 counts, point, then bring the leg down, then repeat with the opposite leg.

Sequence 11 Leg Swings

Start with the back to the barre in first position turnout (with correct body alignment) hands are placed on the barre, the back is in a lifted position to the barre. The hands are slightly relaxed with the arms lifted. For beginners leg swings should start from 1st position.

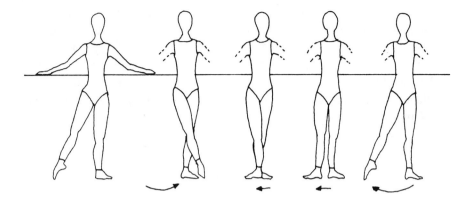

One leg starts crossing over the body in quasi position

- Point

Then returning,

- Brush back turning the heel (ball of the foot first)
- Turnout passing through 5th position
- Then passing through 1st position
- Then pass to a 2nd position and point to a hold.

Then repeating,

- Brush past 1st
- Through 5th
- To 4th
- Point

Repeat this sequence several times.

Repetition of this would depend on the needs of the student. It may be done in 4 counts.

- Count 1   Brush pass
-      2   Brush back
-      3   Brush pass
-      4   Brush back

The transition to the other side starts with pointing the foot, shifting the weight, stepping so your center weight is equal in the 2nd position, then shift the weight, point the left foot, then begin again with the opposite leg.

With the body standing tall, the left foot is out away from the body in 2nd position on point. Cross over, again the heel comes down, point, toe brushes over, and hold. Cross the body quasi, turnback, brush out for 2 counts, then hold passing through. You passthrough from 2nd across the body, to 1st, to 5th across the body, to 4th, turn the toes back, cross going back the way you came and ending in 2nd position.

- Count 1 Cross and point
- 2 Cross open in 2nd
- 3 Cross the body
- 4 Cross the body

Point, step, pull up, change, transition.

Leg swings are taught with several variations: with the straight leg, plie, releve and jumps. Leg swings can be done with turns from the back to the barre, to one hand on the barre facing a new direction (so that the left hand is on the barre) or where the back faces the barre or to the other side where the right hand goes on to the barre and the body faces the barre. These variations and their difficulty depends on the ability and class level.

After the student has understood the leg swings with straight legs (heel does not come off the floor or the knees do not bend). The next variation can be started.

Variation 1

Standing with their back to the barre, the student places his/her right foot to the side. The swings are done through the position above, only now the legs bend at the knee as the foot brushes off the floor. When the leg straightens from plie, the student should continue to releve (quasi, or the foot slightly in a turnout). The counts are the same. This can be repeated on both the right and left side in 4 counts with the transition.

From plie go into releve so that the heel lifts off of the floor. the legs end up in a straight position at the count of 4, brushes down, ends up in a straight position on the count of 4 with the leg away from the body.

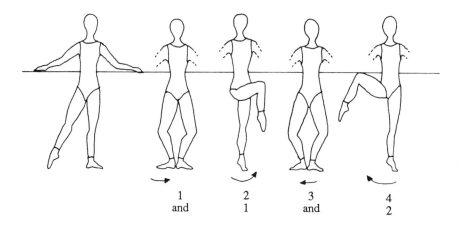

1	2	3	4
and	1	and	2

Variation 2

Still in the count of 4 (depending upon the needs and level of the students), the student can begin with the leg open (either right or left) to its side.

- Count 1   Cross the body

  2   Open

  3   Circle going away from and across the body

  4   On the floor—crossing back across the body

- Hold the leg across the body on count 4 (Quasi, cross the body, attitude, turnout or parallel)

Again, what you are trying to explain to the students would determine whether the legs would be slightly open in a turnout position, attitude position or parallel with the legs straight.

- Count 5   Open away from the body

  6   Cross the body

  7   Open

  8   Circle in towards the body. The leg is up at this point, hold, then bring the leg down. Bring the opposite leg up (switch legs) pull up on the balancing leg.

Then begin again,

- Count 1   Cross the body
  - 2   Open
  - 3   Cross the body and circle
  - 4   Cross the body, hold
  - 5   Swing out
  - 6   Cross the body
  - 7   Open with a complete circle in
  - 8   Hold in open position

This variation can be done in straight leg, plie, and releve. The student always goes back to the center position, carrying the entire weight of the body at the center. The student must step, pull and lift the entire body over the standing leg or the weight will be unbalanced. If not, the student will pull away from the barre, as if to fall with the arms stretched out unequally. The body must always be equally balanced.

A second variation of this movement begins with the left hand on the barre, right foot to the back in slight turnout. The body is pulled up. The right arm (opposite that on the barre) is in Dunham presentation in 2nd position to the side. With the leg in back on point, swing the leg forward in parallel (you have a loose swinging in the hip joint).

- Count 1   Swing forward
  - 2   Swing back. Slight attitude or parallel, depending on the needs of the class. (At level 1 the leg should start in a simple parallel; level 2 students should to into an attitude leg when swinging back).
  - 3   Swing forward
  - 4   Swing back with rotation in hip joint, turning the back to the barre, both hands on the barre
  - 5   Swing across the body
  - 6   Swing open
  - 7   Circle in
  - 8   Lift up with the breath, step, turn the body to a new position
    - front, with the right hand on the barre, bring leg down, turn, left leg in back.

Repeat movement with left leg:

- Count 1   Swing forward
-         2   Swing back
-         3   Swing forward
-         4   Swing back, rotation in the hip joint, back to the barre, both hands on the barre, leg is open-away from the body
-         5   Cross
-         6   Open
-         7   Circle
-         8   Hold

Start the sequence again in plie, then in releve.

Variation 3

Right leg back, left hand on barre, right arm in Dunham presentation, pulling up,

- Count 1   Brush leg through, parallel, plie and straighten
-         3   Plie and straighten, leg is front
-         4   Plie and back, rotate the hip joint, open, back to the barre both hands on the barre
-         5   Cross, plie, straight back
-         6   Open
-         7   Cross, circling out
-         8   Hold, step, change

Repeat movement a total of four complete sets (right side, left side) in straight, plie, releve holding onto the barre, opposite leg in front in balance position. Before executing releve, for a beginning class, keep the students on flat foot or in plie until they understand the total concept of carrying the body with them.

Variation 4

This exercise helps the student to understand the use of the pelvis and the rotation of the hip joint in the socket joint while developing a nice easy swing. The right leg is back, body facing the barre, both hands placed on the barre lightly, feet in slight turnout position, right foot to the back

- Count 1 Swing forward, knee coming up to chest
  2 Swing back
  3 Swing forward
  4 Swing back, swing forward, step, plie, switch to left leg.

or,

- Count 1 Swing forward, knee coming up to chest
  2 Swing back
  3 Swing forward
  4 Swing back, plie to foot and switch

or,

- Start with the foot facing the barre, both hands placed on the barre, slight turn-out, right foot back
- Count 1 Swing forward
  2 Swing back
  3 Swing forward
  4 Swinging back turn the body all the way around, the hip joint rotation should carry you back to the barre with the back up against the barre
  5 Cross the body
  6 Open
  7 Circle
  8 Swing the body all the way back, continuing in a circle clockwise facing back to the barre, hold up, brush down in plie, left leg goes up.
- Repeat sequence facing the barre,
- Count 1 Swing toward barre
  2 Swing back
  3 Swing toward front
  4 Swing all the way around, three-quarters of a turn to the back all the way to the side, the back is facing the barre, both hands are placed lightly on the barre, open
  5 Cross
  6 Open

7   Circle

8   Turn all the way to the back (attitude to the back) facing the barre, leg comes down, switch legs

Leg swing variations can develop into many other movements. You can continue the leg swing variations with up-and-over and hinges to the floor, as well s to leg swings with jumps. Several variations will be expanded upon later.

Sequence 12 Extensions

This exercise begins with the back to the barre, feet in 1st position (parallel), arms are placed lightly on the barre. You begin with the right leg, repeating the sequence with the left leg. Extensions are done to help the student learn how to use the total leg, how to hold the weight of the leg, and how to use the entire torso and the abdominals. Also, the student should be aware of the total placement of the body especially remembering that the upper torso must stay in correct alignment with the head placed between the shoulders, the hips and pelvis elongated and in alignment.

Extensions

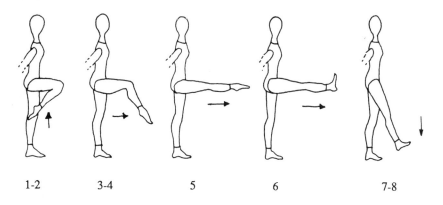

1-2   3-4   5   6   7-8

Begin with the right foot, slightly to the back in a brushing motion going up. Brush the foot up towards the front of the body, keeping the leg bent at the knee.

- Count   1,2,3,4   Foot comes up

         On 4   The knee is bringing the leg up, the lower leg

is dangling from the knee joint (bring the leg up as high as possible but still comfortable).

5   Extend the leg and point the foot. The lower leg must be extended from the knee joint and on the same spacial plane (the thigh and calf is all on one level). If the knee comes up too high on count 4 and the student has to drop the lower leg while extended to another level the leg has been brought up too high.

6   Flex the foot with leg still held up and extended, parallel to the floor. The abdominal muscles are used to hold the leg up.

7,8   Slowly bring the leg down.

The motion is continuous, once understood by the student.

Repeat the movement, in 1st position parallel twice on the right side, then repeat twice on the left side. For a beginning class, when the movement is repeated on the left side, bring the leg back underneath you in a basic standing position. The student would then turn out in a 1st position turnout to repeat the same exercise, hands in the same place, chest and alignment the same but now the legs are working from the turnout position of the thigh muscles, using the abductors to keep the legs turned at the hip joint. The hips should stay down and in place. The right leg will begin to come up, knee first, pointed toe.

- Count 1,2,3,4   Lift, bringing up the knee as high as possible while still being comfortable and the body in proper alignment. The abdominals are holding the leg up, the gluteus maximus is keeping the pelvis under and elongated, hips are down, while using the turnout muscle.

          5   Extend the leg to the side without shifting the torso, foot pointed. This may be difficult for level 1 students until they have a total understanding of their body alignment.

          6   Flex still holding the leg in position

        7,8   Bring leg down to the beginning position

Repeat exercise twice on right and left sides.

This exercise is done with straight leg, as well as with the plie and through plie to releve in a level 1 class. Once the students understand the principle and how to use the total body they can repeat the extensions with transition. The transition moves the body to a new direction, with the left hand on the barre, then the right, making a complete circle in counterclockwise direction. The right hand ends up on the barre and the movement is repeated (total of twice on each side).

- Count 1,2,3,4, Lift
          5 Extend
          6 Flex
          7,8 Bring down

Extensions
Transition

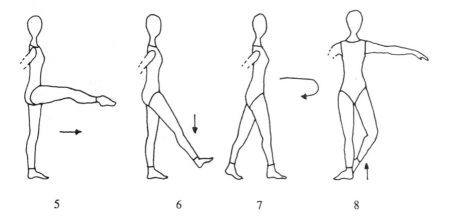

5   6   7   8

- The second time the exercise is done on each leg, transition comes in at count 7 and 8.

Transition: as you come down, the leg is extended out and away from the body. When the foot comes down on eight, the leg is away from the body almost in a 4th position parallel, the student steps toward that foot, bring the entire body toward that foot, then makes a quarter turn to the left. The left hand then extends on the barre, palm down, right arm comes in across the body with a flexed palm holding the elbow straight (total open 4th position parallel). The right leg immediately goes into a triangle shape or a turned out passe with the foot at the ankle. The leg begins to lift. You are now in turn-out. (You have completed two extensions with the back to the barre in parallel.) The transition takes you into the turn-out.

The standing leg (left) is slightly turned out, left hand on the barre, the right leg will now be your active leg.

- Count   1, 2, 3,   Lift up

             4   Hold; turnout, hips are down and under. In this position the instructor should observe from the side view and make sure the hips are not lifted, that the tailbone is long and the abdominals are pulled up, shoulders are not lifted, chin and chest are lifted, arms straight in front.

             5   Extend, hold

             6   Flex, hold

           7,8   Bring down slowly

- Repeat, then go on to the second transition on the count of 7, 8—

Transition: Cross the leg over the left leg, the ball of the foot will touch the floor. On the opposite side of the left foot directly by the side of the metatarsus again pivot staying in the same spacial element that you have. (The students should contain the same distance from the barre when doing transition.) The right hand takes the place of the left, left hand goes in front of the body, straight arm and flexed palm. The leg immediately turns in the triangle position, or turned out passe, right foot to the ankle. The student repeats the exercise. The instructor should again check the body alignment.

- Count   1, 2, 3   Lift up

             4   Hold

             5   Extend with pointed foot

             6   Flex

           7,8   Bring leg down and back behind the right foot that is now the standing and supporting leg.

- This is repeated twice, on the second repeat, the left is brought down stepping behind the right leg going towards the barr, carrying the rest of the body so that you end up in the beginning position.

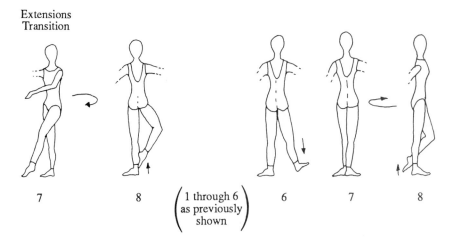

1-2   3-4   5   6

Extensions
Transition

7   8 $\begin{pmatrix} \text{1 through 6} \\ \text{as previously} \\ \text{shown} \end{pmatrix}$ 6   7   8

- Feet in parallel 1st slightly open, both hands on the barre, the chest facing away from the barre the back being closest to the barre.

Repeat the exercise twice on each leg in each direction moving around counterclockwise; in straight legs, plie, plie and straighten, plie to releve. This again depends on the level of the class.

Sequence 13 Leg Whips

Leg Whips is a variation of Extensions. The same process applies, but the leg is actually moving in a swinging motion upwards using the gluteus maximus, hamstring and abdominal muscle to lift the leg. Instead of the knee causing the action, the hamstring and the gluteus is working to start the motion forward. The movement is similar to extensions but is done at a quicker pace, yet very controlled. The quality of movement, uses power from the gluteus and thigh muscle.

There are several objectives of this movement, one is height. Maintain correct body alignment when the leg is at the peak of the movement and as the flexed foot is coming down. The standing leg should stay straight. The student should not bend at the knees at the peak of the movement, but try to stretch the standing leg up as much as possible. The knee goes up to the chest and at the peak of the movement, the foot is flexed. Control on the lowering of the leg is another point of concern. Once at the peak of the movement when the foot is flung up, and the leg starts to descend. The control of the movement is very essential.

This movement is done at an extremely slow tempo. The student may have a tendency to speed up this movement. It is good practice for the instructor to do two tempo variations, extremely slow repeating four times right side, left side, in the transition, turnout left side (four), right side (four), and straight legs, plie and releve. A total of 32 leg whips can be done with the advanced students, after they understand the use of the extension of the leg and the split position that is happening with the standing leg that is supporting the body.

- Count 1   Lift up, knee first in a faster motion, extend
             pointed foot, flex, and come down
- Entire movement is done in one count.

Sequence 14   Up and Over/Pelvic Rolls

Up and over is an exercise that should only be done after the students have perfected the flat-back, fall and recovery, and the pelvic placement exercises. Once these previous exercises are understood, up and over will be less difficult.

Begin with the left hand on the barre, body in a side position. Feet in 1st position parallel, feet slightly turned out. Right arm in Dunham presentation at the hip joint, elbow out. Chin is lifted, inner and outer focus established.

The right arms comes up above the head in Dunham presentation, palm flat, fingers closed thumb in. The breath count will take them up so that they elongate the entire torso. The elbow does not stretch as much as the waist area. The abdominal area lifts up the whole body, as if to add an inch.

Phrase I

- Count 1,2,3,4 Lift up and over, flat back by count 4. Back is in total parallel to the floor, the neck is not broken but is one long spinal position.

Up and Over / Pelvic Rolls

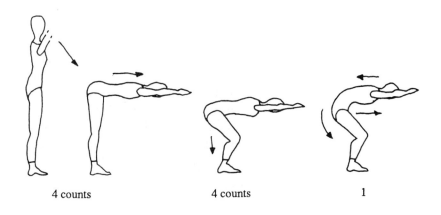

4 counts   4 counts   1

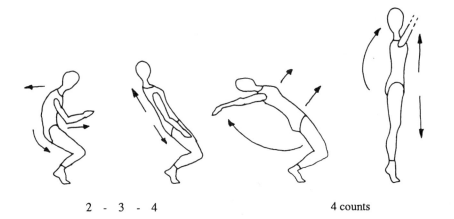

2 - 3 - 4   4 counts

Phrase II

- Count 1,2,3,4   Plie. Knees stay over the toes, hips parallel to the floor, the back and chest stay where they are from the movement above, lowering as the knees lower. The knees are bent, the neck and total spinal column are long, shoulders have not gone up, hand is in the same position, back is long and flat.

Phrase III

- Count 1,2,3,4   Pull through. The pelvis is pulled forward as if there is a string attached to it, as the string is pulled, the pelvis goes straight through, the heels of the feet must come off floor, the back pulls through moving to the back of the body in a hinged position, The knees are bent, the pelvis is tilted forward, and the back becomes an extension of the pelvis The head and the focus is slightly up. The neck is not broken so it is up and forward. The left hand has moved forward, then back to the side.

The right hand has now moved overhead and pulled back with the pelvis that is forward, as if there is a string attached to the side of the hand that is attached to the thigh. This is one motion.

Up to this point, the movement should be repeated several times in a level 1 class before the release of the back.

The next variation of this exercise is to add the release of opening of the chest (the over portion of the exercise). Here the student pushes the pelvis forward more, opening the chest at the same time, not an arch but a thrusting of the pelvis forward (holding the gluteus maximus muscles) and opening the chest at the same time, letting the arm drop down to the floor, and swing behind the head and come forward lifting.

As the students lifts the body up into a standing position in releve, he/she must continue to hold the abdominal and gluteus maximus muscles tight. The students should be reminded to open the chest wide and not to arch.

- In one continuous movement,
- Count 1,2,3,4 Up and over

- Count   1,2   Flat back, plie, parallel hips, pelvis pulled through, back pulled through. Arms pass through, hooking up to the thigh. Long hinge position, hold.
- (As a test the students can release the barre then place hands back on the barre.)
- Pull through, pushing on pressing the pelvis forward more. Chest opens wider, arm drops down to the floor, continuing to circle and bring the chest up. Back up to standing position, releve. Heels come down in the breath phrase of "and" standing and supporting the leg.
- This is repeated twice.
- On the second repeat, the left leg is brought down stepping behind the right leg, which is going toward the barre, carrying the rest of the body so that you end up in the beginning position.

PROGRESSIONS

To start progressions, the students should line up at one end of the room, 3 to 4 people across. When one group has completed a phrase the next group should start 4 or 8 counts behind the first group depending on the particular exercise. The suggested rhythm for beginning progressions Ibo.

Sequence 1   Dunham Walk

The Dunham Walk is done within the understanding of body alignment and placement. The basic walk using the feet is executed with a feeling of a continuous flowing energy through space. The movement begins with the foot stepping away from the body. The right foot (using the toe, ball, arch, and heel). The knee is in plie until the entire foot makes contact with the floor. The weight is shifted to left foot and repeated. This is a gliding movement across the floor that is always in plie. The upper torso is held high and the chin is lifted as the student begins to glide in plie with the feeling of the rhythm coming from within as they move. As they glide and move across the floor, a presence and/or energy level equal to that of being in a processional giving homage must be maintained. The movement should cover space and the student should be in command of that space. The walk is done in a parallel position to the rhythm Ibo.

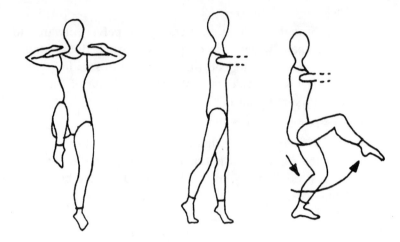

(front)

The arms are in Dunham presentation 2nd position. The arms are parallel to the floor, palms are flat facing the floor, fingers closed, elbows lifted to each side as if the energy is carried upward through the waist. The chest is lifted, shoulders down into the back, chin lifted. The walk starts off gently to the rhythm, stepping to every beat. The object is to hold the hands and arms lifted so that the energy is held consistently as the glide through space is maintained with the entire body. The movement can be started with the left or the right foot. It can be moving backward or forward with any variation that the instructor suggests.

Variation 1 Prance

Once the students have learned the variation above and can stay within the timing of Ibo, they can add a prance step. The prance step uses the whole foot (toe, ball, arch, heel); then the foot comes slightly off of the floor in this pattern:

- Step, plie
- change, step, plie

- step, change, plie
- step, change, plie

The foot comes off of the floor once the prance begins, moving at a fast tempo (in 6/8 time). The prance is similar to a pony step in relation to jazz dance movement and is similar to the prance done in modern dance or ballet with one exceptions; the student glides and plies close to the earth. The whole foot goes down into the ground; the hop lands in plie. The students should imagine themselves doing this prance in dirt rather than on a hardwood floor.

The prance should be done in straight legs, with straight plie, coming forward on the right side, crossing the floor once starting with the right side and coming back across the floor with the left foot.

The arms are in Dunham presentation 2nd position. The arms can also be changed into 5th position above the head, slightly in, then going back to 2nd position.

- Count 1,2,3,4

Prance (single step); arms go down

- Count 1,2,3,4

Prance (single step); arms go above the head

Variation 2 Double Step Prance

Use the same movement as in the variation above, twice on one side:

- Right (toe, ball, arch, heel)
- Lift left, right, lift left, and change
- Repeat

When completing the change, the working leg is straight while the other begins at the toe following through to the ball, arch, heel:

- Right touch left, right touch left, change
- Left touch right, left touch right, change
- Repeat.
- Right ball of foot (flat foot) on the left side, straight knee; right foot is on toe and knee is bent. When you switch the leg goes down straight.

The double step is actually a shift of weight from the right to the left side. Start at one side of the room, lead off with the right leg.

71

When coming back across the floor, the left leg should lead off. The student should become comfortable using either the left or the right side.

Prances can be done across the floor once with right leading off, then with left leading. The double step prance can be done coming back across the floor leading with the right. Alternating steps:

- Single step 4 counts
- Double step 2 counts for each foot (1 set per 4 counts)
- Go back to single step
- Repeat across the floor leading with the right foot across the floor, then leading with the left foot back across the floor.

The double prance step can be repeated with a turn variation and arm movement (the beginning student should do the prance with the arms down or behind their backs). The turn is an inside turn. The upper torso begins to turn inward while the right foot comes slightly to the front.

Starting with the right foot:

- Double step, double step
- Right foot comes slightly in front, turn right
- Double step (right shoulder leading)
- Left foot comes behind and finishes the double step while you step with the right foot to continue the turn. By the time you have taken another double step right and left, you have completed the turn while stepping in towards the body.
- Repeat movement turning in the opposite direction leading off with the left foot

Coming back across the floor (starting with the right) the students can then begin to understand the use of an arm movement. Begin with the double step prance in a forward direction, still doing a turn double right. As they turn with the left foot (the first quarter turn double step), the arms go from 1st position to 2nd position parallel. The right elbow comes in across the body as the left foot begins to move. The elbow moves turns out; when you end up back front, the arm is back in its 1st position parallel moving forward again.

Every time you turn, the left foot begins to work:

- Double right, double left (the arm crosses in front), turns under, turns around, back over and flat—into the starting position)
- Repeat this on the right side

All the way across the floor the same arm is leading in a forward direction. The left arms does not move at all. When repeating on the left side, the right arms does not work at all.

I am sure that there are other variations to the prance step that instructors can come up with using arm movement. Those previously mentioned are the basics.

Sequence 2 Second Position Jumps

Note: Ibo rhythm is still used.

The student starts with a wide 2nd position turnout (that which is used at the barre). Hips are centered, neck sitting balanced between the shoulder blades, proper body alignment, chest lifted, abdominals pulled in, tailbone long and under. Knees opened wide and over the toes, pelvis centered (not hyper-extended). The student jumps forward in this 2nd position contracting forward slightly, to propel the body forward, across the entire floor, using the pelvis and the whole foot. The jump is not high but just skims the floor. The landing is on the toe, ball, arch, and lastly the heel. The power comes from the arch of the foot, ankles and the center which has to stay lifted. The arms are in 2nd position Dunham presentation parallel to the floor, palms down. The objective is to also hold the elbows up bent slightly, while moving across the floor. This is a test of the use of the abdominals to hold the body while at the same time keeping the legs nice and wide with the knees aligned over the toes.

Variation 1

Once the student has completed crossing the floor in this position, a variation to the move can be done by moving the pelvis forward; a very easy forward contraction of the pelvis. The jumps and pelvis contraction should be done in 1 count (move on every beat). For this reason and depending on the skill level of the class, the tempo of Ibo should not be very fast.

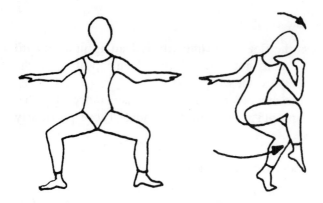

Variation 2

Coming back across the floor, a plie after the jump with a leg lift can be added. This utilizes two exercises from the barre. Thus you would have: jump, jump, lift. The leg comes across the body pausing in a lifted position. Knee is lifted about as high as the waistline, held in a bent position). The standing leg (which, at this point, is the left leg) is bent, right leg is lifted parallel to the floor, foot is pointed, arms are in Dunham presentation.

- Open to 2nd, plie
- Jump into the air
- Jump, plie into the floor
- Jump, lifting with the right leg up off of the floor

It would take 4 jumps to complete the movement in this rhythm:

- Plie, jump; plie, jump, lift.
- Plie, jump; plie, jump lift.

Starting with the right leg, complete the movement then switch to the left leg to repeat the movement. Here, as the leg is coming across the body, each time the leg is lifted and the pelvis is contracted slightly forward (the contraction causes the leg to be lifted). The arms are in Dunham presentation 2nd position. When the right leg is lifted, the left elbow moves towards that leg. Elbow is bent in, palms are facing toward the body. The elbow moves out, back into Dunham presentation 2nd position as the leg goes down. Here you have an opposition movement with the right leg and left arm, and visa-versa. The floor movement starts with the right side and comes back across the floor with the left side.

Variation 3

Once the student has perfected the jump with the leg lift, proceed with the movement across the floor starting on the right side; return on the left side; and an outside turn.

Begin with the right leg, then switch to the left:

- Plie, jump, lift leg
- Plie, jump, lift leg and swing it across while simultaneously swinging the leg around (moving the leg behind the body) landing in 2nd position.

The arms move:

- Lift arm with plie (opposite arm from working leg)
- Arm is down at next plie
- Arms is in at the next jump, turn

Second Position Jumps Variation 3

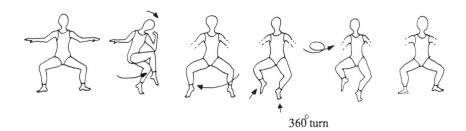

360° turn

In order for students to understand this concept and demonstrate it totally in correct body alignment, they must understand the body alignment moving across the floor first in 2nd position, then across the floor with the pelvic tilt, then across the floor with the leg lift. You cannot teach this exercise without going into the progressions in that order, otherwise the students will not be able to complete the turn while staying low in 2nd position while keeping the back nice and straight.

Being able to do this 2nd position traveling across the floor, turning to the right or left with an outside turn, is one of the Dunham trademarks. Depending on the instructor, an inside turn can also be done. The carriage of the upper torso is in an upright alignment, which helps in accomplishing a perfect landing in 2nd position. This is a difficult exercise and therefore should be repeated several times. This movement is also done in several of the cultural context areas.

Sequence 3   Leap/Rocking Step

This movement is done moving in a forward direction. The student begins in 4th position parallel with the right foot forward and with the weight on the back foot. The weight is then shifted forward to the right foot. The upper torso follows through moving forward.

Back straight, chest and chin lifted. The left leg lifts back, knees bent, toes pointed, and the body is slightly tilted forward. Pelvis is still in line when rocking and the left lifts up.

- Rock forward
- Rock back

When rocking back, the foot is forward (right foot). When you are forward with the chest, the left foot is back. Shift in transition so that the left leg comes forward using the whole foot, toe, ball, arch, heel.

- Rock right (forward), left (back), rock right (forward)
- Kick the left leg through past parallel
- Switch (left foot forward, right arms goes forward across body, left arm goes back)
- Rock left, right, left, swing through, right
- Rock right, left, right, swing through, left

In this movement the leg swings in the parallel position, from the back to the front, adding a rocking motion. Throughout this movement the head does not drop and a nice long line continues through the back. A strong abdominal muscle is needed for this movement to carry the body forward and still control the upper torso.

After the students have understood the barre work and have completed other isolations across the floor along with the other variations,

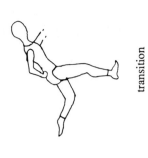

transition

Leap / Rocking Step

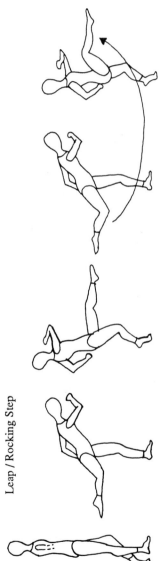

they should have a good concept of their body carriage in this rocking step.

Variation 1 Basic Leg Swing

This movement is a basic leg swing going across the body that the student has learned at the barre. Thus far the student has done the leg swing in a forward direction with the leg staying in a forward parallel position.

Variation 2 Step to the Side

Begin in a slight 4th position with the right or left leg back. The forward and back leg is in a slight turnout position (almost in a 5th position).

- Count 1,2,3
- Rock forward on the right
- Swing left leg back across the body
- Swing to the side—left, right, left
- Swing leg around—left, right, left, right
- Swing leg around across the body, quasi front
- Switch (the knee still comes up parallel to the floor but the leg is swinging around and back to the side front around and back to the side front

The height of this movement can be more exciting to the student than the rocking. Therefore, the height should be monitored closely by the instructor. To the beginning student, the height of the leg is not as important as learning and understanding the mechanics of rocking. Beginning students should not get their legs up too high without totally understanding how to carry their body across the floor in body alignment while rocking. If the student is not careful, the pelvis and the chest can be thrown out of line while trying to get the leg up high.

The intermediate and advanced level student can begin the swing of the leg from the back, to the side and front, making a nice arch and circle.

Variation 3 Adding a Turn

- The body is turned so that it rocks forward
- Right, left, right, swing

Leap / Rocking Step Variation 3 - Adding a Turn

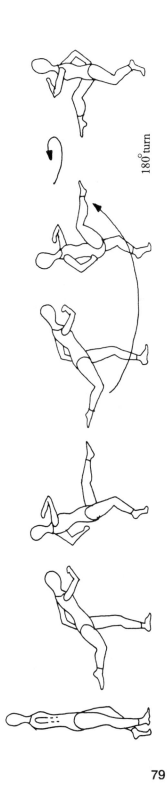

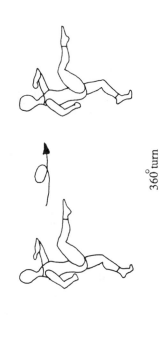

180° turn

360° turn

79

- left, right, left; change direction
- Still moving forward, change the direction from which you came
- Right, left, right, swing
- Left, right, left, swing right
- Change direction in which you are going across the floor
- Right, left, right, change
- Left, right, left, swing right
- Change direction to which you are going away from
- Right, left, right, left
- Left, right, left, change

Sequence 4 Traveling Isolations

Note: This movement can be done to the rhythm that the instructor chooses. If already working with Ibo, you may want to continue in that rhythm.

Sequence 4 - Traveling Isolations

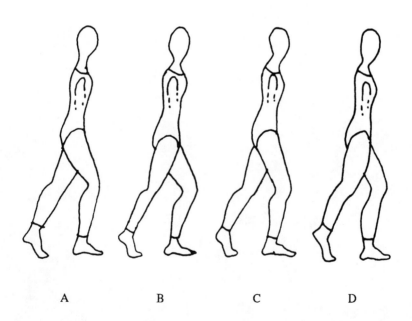

A   B   C   D

Traveling isolations should move from the head, through the shoulders, chest and hips. The basic concept is to give the students an understanding of how to move and isolate a certain part of the body in conjunction with locomotion movement and to move that part of the body across the floor. The beginning isolations should be done standing in one place working each body part. Now we begin to put those body parts on top of a rhythm moving through space.

Begin in plie, stepping with a flat foot In plie, the student gets the feeling of being in contact with the earth as opposed to flying in space and losing control. The rhythm base is found through the pelvic and abdominal areas, knees bent, using the floor.

Head

Moving (stepping) across the floor, isolate the head moving it down and back (chin should touch the chest on the down movement of the head).

Head

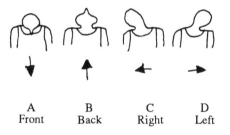

| A | B | C | D |
| Front | Back | Right | Left |

Returning across the floor, isolate the head, moving it side to side (chins goes to each shoulder).

Head Variations

Then add motion variations of down, back, right, left, or circling.

Circles

With circles the step can change to

• Side

• Together

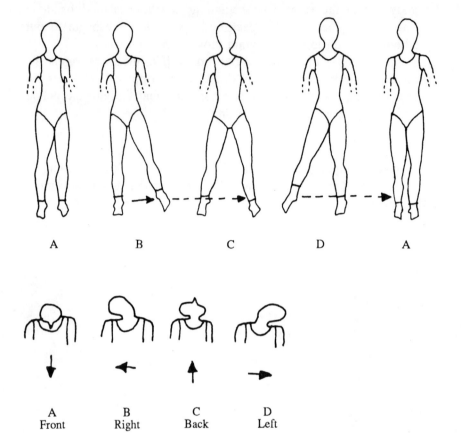

A	B	C	D	A

A Front	B Right	C Back	D Left

- Side
- Touch
- or, looking to the side which you are moving
- Circle
- Circle
- Hold

Head Quivers
Head quivers is shaking the head quickly to the side.

Head Quivers

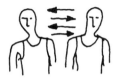

Pecking

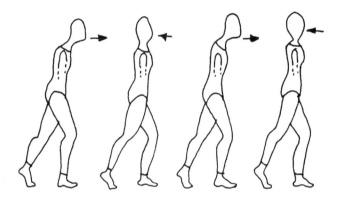

Pecking
Pecking is a forward and back motion that can be added.

Body Turns
To add a body turn, when turning right

- Step left
- Step right
- Touch left (turn completed)
- Turning left
- Step left
- Step right
- Step left
- Touch right

Head circles are done with this movement.

Each head isolation can be done separate or with variations added while going across the floor. For example:

- Count 1,2,3,4
- Down, back, right, left
- Circle and right, hold
- Circle and left, hold
- Quivering (2,3,4,)
- Peck front and back
- Peck front and back

Moving in the same direction, these isolations can be done

- Count 1,2,3,4
- Walk forward, head moving
- Down and back
- Down and back

Body Turns

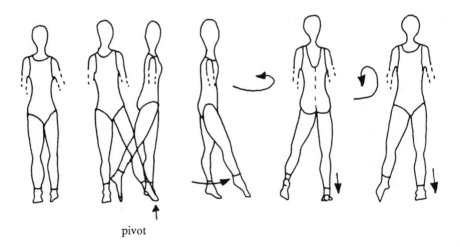

pivot

or,

- Walk forward, head moving
- Right side, left side,
- Right side, left side

or,

- Head circles with a change in step moving to the side
- Step right, step left
- Step right, and hold

or,

- Turning
- Step right
- Step left—turning right
- Step right
- Touch left and hold
- Step left,
- Step right—turning left
- Step left
- Touch right and hold

or,

- Move forward with the fast quiver

or,

- Peck
- Front and back
- Front and back

Shoulders

Still moving in a forward direction each of the following movements can be done with the shoulders:

- Count 1,2,3,4
- Shoulders move up and down

Shoulders

or,

- Both shoulders go front and back

or,

- Shoulders move in opposition
- Right and back

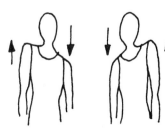

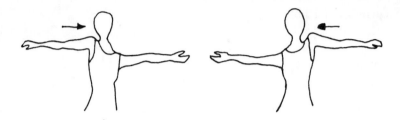

- Left and back

or,

- Quiver shoulders forward
- Right and left

or,

- Move shoulders in opposition
- Right and left

or,

- Circle the shoulders back with the foot in 4th position standing base step, stepping backwards with the right foot as lead
- Count 1, 2, 3   Right foot and right shoulder moves back
           4   Right foot and shoulder comes front
              Switch to left foot and shoulder
              Repeat movement

or,

- Move forward switching right and left shoulders

or,

- Move backward switching right and left shoulders

or,

- Center, move back, center

Use as many variations in this shoulder movement as you can think of. A change in levels can also be made:

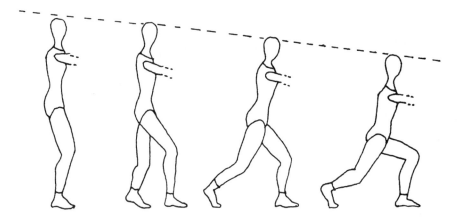

- Forward and back, repeat

or,

- Circle forward, repeat 3 times
- Stop in 4th position parallel
- Circle down (lower body into plie while circling the shoulders back simultaneously
- Plie, come up (stretching legs)
- Circle forward and up, repeat 3 times
- Switch to left foot
- Alternate feet—left, right, left right
- Circle down (left foot back and left shoulder circling)
- Come up, shoulders moving forward
- Switch legs

Chest

Move the isolation down to the chest

- Chest comes forward and back, repeat
- Chest moves side to side, repeat

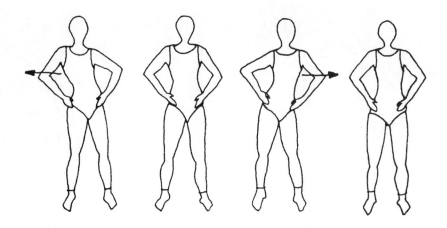

These chest isolations can be done with the feet moving in a simple walk. The chest can go into a body roll (almost a Damballa) using the 4th position standing base:

- Roll the chest down, and up
- Move forward, front and back
- Repeat motion
- Count 1,2,3,4
- Stop and roll down (one continuous motion)
- Count 1,2,3,4
- Come up
- Count 1,2,3,4
- Moving the chest in the same direction
- Walk to the side, left
- Right
- Left

Hips

From the chest move down the body to the hips

- Count 1,2,3,4
- Step forward, contract pelvis forward

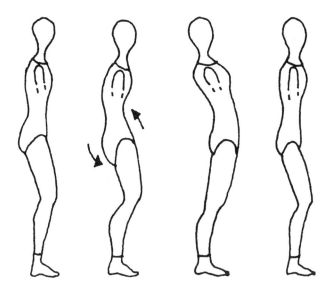

- Step back, contract pelvis back
- Repeat the movement

or,

- Contract pelvis front, step, contract (alternating feet)

The arm movements are controlled by the instructor. Many of the movements can be with the arms hanging down to the side. In this way the students can concentrate on the part of the body that is being isolated.

When doing the pelvic contractions, the arms may come up with the hip that is doing the contraction; also you can have opposition.

- Right hip forward, left arm forward in bent position, palm facing up

Across the floor you may do the pelvic contraction going in a forward direction. Coming back across the floor you may alternate a front and back direction. Then the hip may go to the side. In this movement the standing base can be a wide 2nd with one foot flat and

Hips

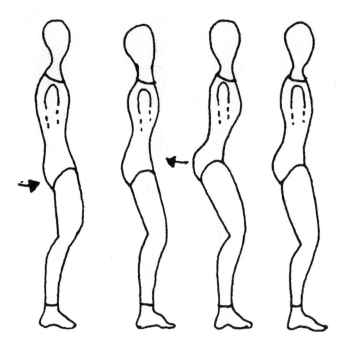

Hips

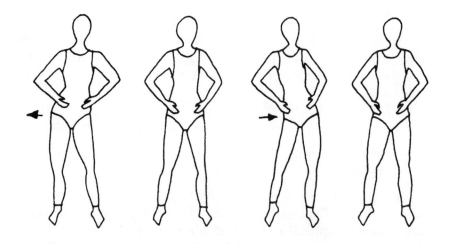

90

the other up on the ball of the foot. This gives you freedom to move the hips.

The hips move front and back in one motion to the side. Everytime the hips move front, pick up the front foot; when hips move back, pick up the back foot, then put it down.

Hips - with Bent Knees

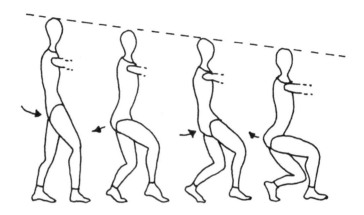

- Lift up the foot
- Bend the knee
- Pelvis lifts up
- Put it down
- Back foot moves up
- Put it down
- Back foot move in
- Contract forward
- Contract back (pull hips out alignment)
- Pull other foot in closer to the standing leg
- Right, pull in left (pelvis is contracted back)
- Contract forward (in plie) (right foot is flat)
- Contract back (left leg is up on the ball of the foot)
- Switch to the left side

Variation 1 Hip Circles

This same base foot can be used in the hip circles. In this movement you contract forward, hip circles front, side and back in one continuous motion. The feet are flat plie; the back foot (ball of the foot) is flat in plie when circling back.

Hip Circles

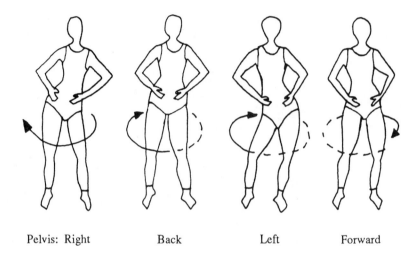

| Pelvis: Right | Back | Left | Forward |

- Contract forward
- Circle forward
- Circle back
- Repeat
- Come in and contract

Here is an isolation progression variation that should be followed in sequence:

- Hips go front and back, repeat
- Hips go side and front, repeat

or,

- Move to the side with the pelvis going front and back, then add circles

Variation 2 Hip Circle with Turns

The same turns used with the head, shoulder, or chest isolations can be added to the hip circles (the outside turn is easier than the inside turn).

The rhythmic variations you can add to this are endless. This is a very important aspect of traveling isolation. The rhythm of the hips can be going to one rhythm while the head moves to another rhythm. The feet can move at a slow pace and the hips at a fast pace. The rhythm of isolation depends on the instructor. Here the student learns to understand and move to the rhythmic variations.

Once the students can perfect the isolation of one body part with the feet moving, they can go back and add two isolations together (i.e., shoulder and head, hip and head, chest and head).

Progressions in Cultural Context

Beckford states that progressions is "the term used for a movement pattern done across the floor." Not only are progressions simple movement patterns done across the floor but they are the students' opportunity to increase their ability to perfect the movement that they have done at the barre or isolation from stationary center floor. The student combines these movement combinations in the sequences which the teacher directs him/her and begins to move across the floor from one designated starting point to another. The student then must put it all together; rhythm, style and quality of movements. The centering, focusing, alignment, and attention must all come to a point of intersecting for total execution of the movement phrase.

Progressions in Cultural Context is built around the same basic principle of simple progressions, moving from one point in the room to another. The difference is that now specific rhythm forms are used, rhythms that reflect a cultural heritage of a specific cultural group. The main cultural influence that Miss Dunham uses is that of Haiti, but it is not the only rhythm style that appears. These specific rhythms usually have specific dance steps that accompany them, and these steps usually reflect the basic concept of that dance or why that dance is performed.

This aspect of the technique is a direct influence of Miss Dunham's work as an Anthropologist and her belief in synchronization. Her research done in Haiti gives the basic information and concepts for Progression in Cultural Context. Damballa, Yanvalou, Zepalues and others are specific rhythms or dieties that are repre-

93

sented in the vodum ceremonies or the basic celebration of everyday life in the Haitain, Martinique, Jamaica, Cuba, or other West Indies cultures. The other area of representation is Jazz dance. Miss Dunham recognized the rhythm and movement style connection between Jazz dance of the African-American cultural in the United States and that of the Islands of the West Indies.

There were no dance techniques that would give Miss Dunham and her Dancers the unique style, strength, and rhythm needed to perform her choreography with the authenticity and the quality that was needed. Progression in cultural context is the fusion of what she needed to train her dancers. This type of technique helps give the audience the accurate visual perception of the dances. The early technique work at the barre, center floor, isolation, and basic progression are the foundations for the development of movement in cultural context, or movement that has been created specifically for performance by the choreographer.

Miss Dunham's descriptions of several of these rhythms or dances were first listed in her book *Dances of Haiti*, or have been documented in descriptions of specific choreographies that were done for stage.

Damballa

Damballa is the Serpent god in the Vaudum religion. The movement that represents this particular deity is a slow undulating movement of the torso. The movement breakdown has been described throughout the foundation of the techniques from the barre work to center floor as *body rolls*. If the student has already perfected this movement concept, then the execution of Damballa and its variation will be simple.

The upper torso is moving in continuous fluid motions that move throughout the entire spine.

> Yonvalou, the dance of humility and assurance. This dance to the serpent Damballa, the Haitian vaudun god, begins at the base of the spine by contracting or tucking under the hips in an upward tilt. Like a ripple in a pool of water, the movement starts to follow up the spine to the neck and finishes at the neck and head only to start again in the hips in an unbroken circuit. (Beckford pg. 52)

This movement does not stop, so one is not aware of where the movement begins or ends. The position of the legs, knees and feet as the upper body is moving through the motion, can use several variations; the knees always bend within the rhythmic pattern of the movement. The feet move in a step-together-step from side to side, forward

94

and backwards, in circles, slow or fast. The movement can also add level changes from high to low, and variations on tempo: fast, slow or very slow.

Yanvalou

Yanvalou is the Religious Dance that honors Damballa. Yanvalou has a specific rhythm that is played. This rhythm is usually in 3/4 or 6/8 time. The movement concept is the same as Damballa, undulating movements of the torso. This undulating free flowing movement can manifest itself in any part of the body, arms, hands, hips as well as the torso. The student should be able to do the movement so that an observer would not be able to see where the movement starts or ends. The movement should always be continuous. The tempo of the movement is usually set by the drummers. The variations on this dance are many. The movement can travel in any direction, use all levels possible and any body parts. Even within a traditional ceremony itself, the level of improvisation is unlimited.

Zepaules

Zepaules is a dance of the voudum done for the deity. Legba and others. Legba is the god that is the gatekeeper. This particular dance is a perfect example of why Miss Dunham developed Isolation and the need for her dancers to be able to perfect such movement styles. Zepaules is a movement that uses rapid shoulder isolation. Thus keeping the other parts of the body still, the main emphasis is on the shoulders moving in unison, pushing downward. The shoulder movement is of a percussive quality that pushes downward, then up with the feeling of the energy going through the back of the body.

The movement of the feet accompanying the body is the same rapid tempo as the shoulders. The movement is usually small steps taken in a forward direction, with knees bent slightly. The feet leave the floor in a flat foot position lifting off and returning the same.

Congo Paillette

A dance done with both men and women approaching each other "with sexual intent."* The rhythm of this dance is usually of a medium tempo. The use of bent knees, isolation of hip and chest, body parts are the main focus point. The dancers work as couples, and their eye focus is on each other. The movement can be taken in a circular pattern or in a follow-the-leader approach. The couple moves away from each other but still looks at each other, then moves in a forward direction, then back to each other.

Petro

Petro is a cult of the Haitian voudum, usually considered violent or negative. Within the context of progression and dance technique, Petro is usually a fast tempo rhythm, with a quality of urgency in the movement. The movements that are done are a combination of isolation of the upper torso and the feet doing several styles, Ibo, Mahi, even the possibility of basic prance step. Here the rhythm is the important factor and the students' ability to be able to execute movement phrase within the rhythm is of importance.

Banda

The banda is officially a funeral dance and may be private and ceremonial, with cult supervision, or free, secular, and public, depending entirely on the wishes of the family of the deceased. (Dunham *Dance of Haiti* Pg. 10)

It is a symbolization of man's rebirth as he rises from the dead. It is man's second life. (Williams *Haiti Dance pg. 11)*

For the purpose of learning Dunham technique, the student here is more concerned with the application and execution of the rhythmic pattern. The rhythm is moderate in tempo, with fints or breaks throughout. The drummers control the movement phrase as to where these breaks may come. The basic movement style is a percussive isolation movement coming spontaneously throughout the body on the fints or breaks of the drum. The feet carry the body forward or on a serpentine direction forward, sometimes moving backwards or even turning around in a circle, then continuing on in the forward direction. The body is moving in an abandonment quality, and the movement breaks take on a sexual or poking fun at the nature of man.

Mahi (my-ee)

The Mahi can really be called the dance of the feet. (Williams pg. 9)

Mahi is a fast rhythmic tempo, with very percusive movements. The knees are bent with the upper torso being carried in a stately manner with movement variation from isolation to smooth undulation movement, as body rolls. The feet are the main focus of this dance; with flat feet, one foot is picked up (one at a time) moving forward, then to the back in an arc motion. The other leg never leaves the plie

96

position at the knee. The same foot is then placed down in the back of the support foot, almost in a straight line behind it. This is all done in a constant motion, moving in a forward direction, with the movement alternating from one side to the other. This particular movement combines poly rhythm with the upper torso at a different tempo and quality of movement. This is also one of the most difficult movements to perfect or teach. One should give her/himself the opportunity to have hands-on experience of this particular exercise.

Other African Rhythmic Styles

There are many variations and dance styles and rhythmic patterns that can be used for the student to perfect and learn progressions in cultural context. Other areas that Miss Dunham has created out of her research for her Professional company and for the present Children Workshop include: Rhythms and styles of Congo/Comparsas of Cuba, Samba and Frefro of Brazil and Argentina. The concepts are endless and varied. This is where a teacher or student of the Dunham Technique needs to expand his/her knowledge beyond the textbook, seek out and find hands-on experience of dances within their cultural context. To leave this to the interpretation of the written word only would be too simplistic, negating the wealth and excitement of the spirit of a culture.

DUNHAM CHAKRA ADAGIO SEQUENCE

The Chakra sequence was introduced to the participants of the 1988 Seminar by Miss Dunham. As in other Exercises of Dunham Technique it has many variations, using the body in the seated or standing position. Only the original seated position is described in this text.

The Chakra sequence shows a religious and cosmological influence in Dunham's work. This influence is also apparent in her work with the Africans of the diaspora throughout the Americas. This influence appears in many of the progressions in cultural context and her personal approach in teaching a class.

Chakra

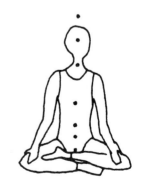

7
6
5
4
3
2
1

Africans brought with them as a part of their cultural heritage a cosmology and a belief system that appears throughout their movement expression. Often times this sense of relationship to the universe and their belief system would bring about a high level of spiritual enlightenment if learned and practiced. "The word Chakra is Banskrit, and signifies a wheel" (C.W. Leadbeater 1927 p1). It too is used as part of movement expression within a cultural context to reach a level of enlightenment.

There are seven Chakra points. Each one represents a specific area of energy and mental understanding of one's self and their position within the universe. The mental or enlightenment aspect is not discussed in this text. This should not be negated if it is going to be taught. The author suggests that further study should be done on and explanation of Chakras through other sources.

- **Chakra One:** is the root or base Chakra. It is physically located at the base of the spine.
- **Chakra Two:** is physically located near the sacral and prostate area.
- **Chakra Three:** is located behind the naval near the solar plexus.
- **Chakra Four:** is the Heart Chakra.
- **Chakra Five:** is located in the throat and thyroid area.
- **Chakra Six:** is located in the center of the skull (the third eye).
- **Chakra Seven:** is the crown chakra, above the head.

For the Dancer, the Chakras represent the ability to control each point as they represent the energy force of movement application. The mastering of these energy points would mean ultimate control of one's body as it is propelled through space.

Chakra Sequence
- Starting in a seated position with the legs crossed in front of the body (Lotus Position).
- The spine is erect, knees bent with the legs open out to both sides of the body (turnout at the hip joint), the feet are crossed at the ankles.

- The arms are suspended loosely at the shoulder joint with the hands resting on the knees, palms facing upward in a cupped position.
- The eyes are closed and the focus is inward. The only conscious sounds that the student should be aware of are the drums and the voice of the teacher.

Starting in this position, the student should then be directed to concentrate on each Chakra point, from the first through the seventh. Starting with a conscious application of breathing, the student should add a contracting and releasing motion of the body in an upwardly moving direction through each Chakra area. This movement should be developed in a pattern where the energy is a smooth continuous flow, moving throughout the body without stopping. When the Seventh Chakra is reached, the movement returns to the First and continues without a break in motion

Each one of these movement phrase through the body should be set to a rhythmic pattern. This rhythmic pattern is set by the teacher and accompanied by drums. The sound that is brought forth from the drums should be *deep, strong* tones. These tones should be strong enough to generate a resonance of sound which will carry the vibration throughout the body, thus creating the feeling state for the student of being one with the drums.

The movement pattern continues with the First Chakra: Contraction then release of the buttocks.

- Moving to the Second Chakra, stretching through the spine to the Third Chakra continuing to stretch to the upper spine, then the body begins to lean forward in a angle position towards the floor.
- As the movement reaches the Fourth Chakra, the movement flow is proceeding through the torso, the hands turn over and palms are placed on the floor (the hands are still slightly cupped).
- As the Fifth Chakra is reached (focus is on the throat area), the body is still tilted towards the floor the hands move forward with the body.
- The arms are outstretched on the floor in order to assist in controlling the body downwards to the floor.

- At the sixth Chakra (the forehead is the point of focus), the body is reaching towards the floor, the arms are still outstretched above the head.
- The Seventh Chakra is reached at this point; the legs are still crossed and the hip joints are open to a full turned out position, placed on the floor.

The next part of this sequence will allow the student to come to full standing position.

- As the Student is lying with the front of the body facing the floor, legs crossed, arms outstretched with the weight of the body held in the chest and abdominal area. The body is then released onto the floor. The legs are released slowly, stretching below the torso.
- The right foot starts the next movement, carrying the leg across the back of the body reaching in an attitude position; place the foot on the floor allowing the body to follow the leg into a sitting position. As the body is carried the other leg bends and the foot is placed on the floor.
- In this seated position, one arms is stretched out in front of the body, the other towards the back. The hand in back is placed on the floor to assist in the motion to carry the body forward.
- The pelvic area is where the motion is initiated, causing the body to move forward, followed by the abdominal area, the chest, the hand in the back pushes, the head follows and the body comes to a standing position.
- Reversing the direction, the student returns to the floor with one arm reaching towards the floor, the other forward on a high diagonal level.
- The body is being held through the pelvis and torso, the head leads as the body lowers to the floor, sliding the body onto the floor in a straight position.
- The legs then fold back into the Lotus position, the movement continues in a slow undulating flow, causing the body to reverse itself back into the sitting position.
- The body is now back to the very first starting position. The movement sequence is repeated on the other side.

Once the sequence is accomplished on the opposite side of the body, the Chakra Adagio exercise has been completed.

This exercise has been most frequently used by Miss Dunham at the beginning of a class. In many instances, it has constituted the entire class period. I have applied the exercise at the close of a class session. However it is applied, whether at the beginning or the end of a class session, or even at other times during a sessions, the overall objective is the same. And that is, to focus and draw upon the multiple energy centers of the body.

Conclusion

In writing this limited text on Dunham Technique, it has been my purpose to prepare a simple, but thorough text which can be used by both teachers and students of dance in the most basic and fundamental applications. Obviously I have relied upon many sources. My prime source has been my personal involvement with Miss Dunham and The Dunham Technique Seminars. Other sources have been acknowledged throughout the book.

The theories and methodologies which I've discussed, and which evolved from ideas and concepts developed by Miss Dunham, are both learnable, and transferable. It has been my devotion to this belief that has reinforced my commitment to writing this text. I've stated at the beginning that I felt it was important to document and preserve that aspect of the Dunham legacy which constitutes to me, in my own personal growth and development, to have had the kind of exposure to experience, which working in the Dunham seminars and teaching Dunham Technique has brought me. Such experience has enhanced the quality of my work in the classroom and the dance studio, as well as improving upon my technique as a performer in earlier years.

There is no doubt in my mind that you will benefit from this sharing of my exposure to experience, provided you become willing to devote yourself to the personal practice of the Technique in dancing and in teaching.

Individuals at all levels of achievement in the art of dance, teachers and students alike, can benefit from The Technique as set forth in this printed text. Keep in mind, though, that Dunham Technique, while it consists of a system of identifiable and learnable and transferable qualities, is always subject to continuous change and variation.

The reason, of course, is because of the current impact that is still being made by Miss Dunham as she continues to conduct Dunham Technique sessions in East St. Louis and throughout the country and the world.

Because of what I and countless others have gained from being involved in The Dunham Technique experience, I encourage you to experience Dunham Technique—its Theories, Methodologies, and Philosophy in your life!

References

Aschenbrenner, Joyce
1981 *Katherine Dunham: Reflections on the Social and Political Contexts of Afro-American Dance.* New York: Congress on Research in Dance.

Beckford, Ruth
1979 *Katherine Dunham A Biography.* New York: Marcel Dekker.

Biemiller, Ruth
1969 *Dance: The story of Katherine Dunham.* New York.

Clark, Veve and Margaret B. Wilkerson (editors)
1978 *Kaiso! Katherine Dunham An Anthology of Writings.* Berkeley: University of California.

Dunham, Katherine
1959 *A Touch of Innocence.* New York: Harcourt, Brace & World, Inc.

1968 The Performing Arts of Africa. First World Festival of Negro Arts: Colloquium. Speech given.

1969 *Island Possessed.* Garden City, N.Y.: Doubleday & Company, Inc.

1974 *Syllabus on Dunham Technique.* Southern Illinois University.

1983 *Dances of Haiti.* Los Angeles: Center for Afro-American Studies. University of California at Los Angeles.

1971 *Journey to Accompong.* Westport, Connecticut: Negro Universities Press.

1941 Thesis Turned Broadway. *California Arts and Architecture. In Kaiso! Katherine Dunham An Anthology of Writings.* by Clark and Wilkerson 1978. Berkeley: University of California.

1976 "Dance As Cultural Art and Its Role In Development." Paper delivered by Ms. J. Stovall, Dakar, Senegal. In *Kaiso! Katherine Dunham An Anthology of Writings* by Clark and Wilkerson. 1978. Berkeley: University of California.

1941 Form and Function In Primitive Dance. *Educational Dance Journal* 4, no. 4 (October 1941)

1972 *Reflections on Survival.* Paper presented at MacMurray College Commencement Address, Jacksonville, Illinois.

1986 *Minefield.* Unpublished manuscript.

1985   *Conversion with Katherine Dunham.* Dunham Technique Seminar, taped session.

Leadbeater, C. W.
1987   *The Chakras.* Wheaton, Illinois: The Theosophical Publishing House.

Smith, M. D. and Fritz Frederick
1986   *Inner Bridges: A Guide to Energy Movement and Body Structure.* Atlanta, Georgia: Humanics Limited.

Thompson, Roy
1978   Focal Rites: New Dance Dominions. In *Kaiso! Katherine Dunham An Anthology of Writings*, by Clark and Wilkerson. Berkeley: University of California.

Thompson, Robert Farris
1983   *Flash of the Spirit: African & Afro-American Art & Philosophy.* New York: Random House.

Yarborough, Lavinia Williams
       Haiti-Dance. Germany: Bronners Druckere; Frankfurt aur Main, 1958.

Note: Many of the research findings that appear in this text are from personal interviews and discussions with Miss Dunham, and on her recommendation, the reading or viewing of her private collection of Papers, Books, Films and Video Tapes.

APPENDIX

KATHERINE DUNHAM
CURRICULUM VITAE

Born

Chicago, Illinois to Albert Millard Dunham and Fannie Guillaume Dunham, school principal; mother Annette Poindexter Dunham, school teacher, Chicago, Illinois. Father choral singer in Umbrian Glee Club. Owner, cleaning and dyeing establishment.

Married

July 10, 1949 to John Thomas Pratt, theatrical designer, one daughter, Marie Christine.

Address

532 North 10th St., East St. Louis, Illinois 62201. Residence Katherine Dunham, B.P. 1283, Port au Prince, Haiti, West Indies.

Education

Graduate of Joliet Township High School and Junior College, University of Chicago, Ph.B., Graduate studies in Social Anthropology; Masters Degree Candidate-Science, University of Chicago, *"Dances of Haiti: Their Social Organization, Classification, Form and Function"*.

Honorary Degrees

Doctor of Humane Letters, MacMurray College, Jacksonville, Illinois, 21 May 1972.

Doctor of Literature, Atlanta University, Atlanta, Georgia, 16 May 1977.

Doctor of Fine Arts, Westfield State College, Westfield, Massachusetts, 26 May 1979.

Doctor of Fine Arts, Brown University Providence, Rhode Island, 4 June 1979.

Doctor of Fine Arts, Dartmouth College of Hanover, New Hampshire, 10 June 1979.

Doctor of Fine Arts, Washington University, St. Louis, Missouri, 22 May 1981.

Doctor of Fine Arts, Southern Illinois University, Edwardsville, 10 June 1983.

Doctor of Laws, Lincoln University, Pa., May 6, 1984.

Doctor of Fine Arts, Howard University, Washington, D.C. May 12, 1984.

Memberships

- American Guild of Musical Artists, Board of Governors, 1943–49
- American Guild of Variety Artists
- American Federation of Radio Artists
- American Society of Composers and Publishers
- Sigma Epsilon Honorary Women's Scientific Fraternity
- Royal Society of Anthropology, London
- Screen Actors Guild
- Actors' Equity
- The Authors Guild, Inc.

Experience

Theatre

- Chicago Opera, Guest Star 1933–36
- Chicago World's Fair Choreographer/performer, 1934
- Concert, Rex Theatre, Port au Prince Haiti, 1937
- *Run Lil Chillun,* Chicago production, Choreographer
- Goodman Theatre, Chicago 1938
- *Pins and Needles,* New York, Choreographer, 1939
- *Tropics and Le Jazz* Hot, New York, 1939
- *Cabin in the Sky,* New York and tour, 1939–41, Los Angeles and West Coast, 1942
- *Tropical Review,* New York and tour, 1943–44
- *Carib Song,* New York, 1945

- *Bal Negre,* New York and tour, 1946, Mexico, 1947. Transcontinental tour, 1948
- Caribbean Rhapsody, London, Paris, Europe, 1948–49. South America, 1950–51; Europe, North Africa, 1952–53; United States, Mexico, 1953; Germany, Europe, 1954; South America, 1954–55; Mexico, 1955; Greek Theatre, U.S., Broadway, 1955–56; /australia, New Zealand, 1956–57; Far East, 1958; Europe, Near East, Argentina, 1959,19660
- *Bamboche,* U.S. tour, 1962; New York, 1963

Motion Picture House Presentations
- Fox Theatre, Los Angeles, 1942
- Roxy, New York, 1946
- Adams, Newark, 1947
- Golden Gate, San Francisco, 1948–49
- United Artist, Los Angeles, 1949
- Carib, Kingston, Jamaica, 1951
- Opera Buenos Aires, 1954
- Windsor Palace, Barcelona, Spain, 1956
- Apollo, New York, 1963–64–65

Motion Picture/Personal Appearances
- Carnival of Rhythm, Hollywood's first dance film in color, 1939
- Star Spangled Rhythm, 1941
- Stormy Weather, 1943
- Casbah, 1949
- Botta e Riposta, Paris, 1952
- Mambo, 1954
- Musica en la Noche and others, Mexico, 1957
- Other films: Germany, Argentina, Japan, Rome

Night Clubs and Hotels
- College Inn, Sherman Hotel, Chicago
- Chez Paree, Chicago
- Mark Hopkins, Fairmont and La Fiesta, San Francisco

- Rancho Vegas and Sahara, Las Vegas, 1947 & 1959
- Mapes Hotel, Reno
- Lake Tahoe and Palm Springs
- Ciro's, Hollywood, 1947–1948
- Little Trocadero, Hollywood
- Versailles, Mexico City
- Sporting d'Ete and Sea Club, Monte Carlo
- Casinos in Nice, Cannes, Juan les Pins, Menton, Biarritz, Arcachon, La Boule, Annecy, others
- La Martinique, New York
- Chalfonte, Atlantic City
- Latin Quarter and Eden Rock, Miami
- Benibashi, Tokyo, 1957
- Mar-del-Plata, Argentina

Open Air Theatres and Arenas
- Theatre de Verdure: Monte Carlo, Nice, Cannes
- Marseilles Arenas: Dax, Acho, Lima
- Roman Amphitheatres: Mines, Arles
- Madison Square Garden, New York
- Port au Prince, Haiti
- Greek Theatre, Los Angeles
- Hollywood Bowl, Santander, Spain, Mexico City
- Bull Ring Arenas: Lima, Peru; Bogota, Colombia

Opera Houses
- Chicago Civic Opera
- Colon of Buenos Aires
- San Francisco
- Santiago de Chile
- Palacio de Bellas Artes, Mexico
- Kiel Auditorium, St. Louis

Choreography and Staging

Films
- Star Spangled Rhythm, Hollywood, 1941
- Pardon My Sarong, Hollywood, 1952
- Native Son, Argentina, 1951
- Mambo, Rome, 1954
- Green Mansions, Hollywood, 1959
- The Bible, Rome, 1959
- Others: Mexico, Germany, South America, Japan

Opera
- Aida, Metropolitan, New York, 1964
- Faust, Southern Illinois University, Carbondale, 1965
- Treemonisha, Atlanta, 1972; Wolftrap Farm Park for the Performing Arts, Vienna, Virginia, 1972; Southern Illinois University, Carbondale, 1972

Theatre Direction
- Tropical Pinafore, Chicago, 1939
- New Version, Pins and Needles, 1939
- I Hear America Singing, New York, 1939
- Deux Anges, Paris, 1965
- Ciao, Rudi, Rome, 1965
- San Remo Festival, New York, 1966
- Ballet National, Dakar, Senegal, 1966–67
- Dream Deferred, Southern Illinois University, East St. Louis, IL, 1968
- Ode to Taylor Jones, Southern Illinois University, East St. Louis, IL, 1968
- Rags and Such, Wolftrap Farm Park for the Performing Arts, Vienna, Virginia, 1975

Television
- First hour-long American Spectaculars, telecast NBC, 1939
- Spectaculars, BBC, London, 1952
- Spectaculars, National Television, Paris, 1952–53

- Spectaculars, Buenos Aires, 1955
- Spectaculars, Toronto, CNS, 1956
- Debut Australian television, Sidney, 1957
- Others; T.V. appearances, Mexico, Germany
- Interview and Panel shows
- Esso World Theatre, New York, 1954
- Personal appearances, 1969
- Interview, The Dick Keefe Show 4/CBS, St. Louis, 22 January 1978
- Interview the McNeil-Lehrer Report, nationwide, PBS, 17 July 1978
- Dance in America Series, PBS, nationwide; Divine Drumbeats: Katherine Dunham and Her People, April 1980
- Interview, Eye on St. Louis, 4/CBS, St. Louis, October 1981

Lectures
- University of Chicago, 1937
- Yale University, 1939
- Mexico, Bellas Artes: Acta Anthropologica, 1947
- Royal Anthropologica Society, London, 1948
- Royal Anthropological Society, Paris, Palais dc Chaillot, 1949
- Brazil, 1950; New Zealand, 1957; Salzburg, 1965
- First World Festival of Negro Arts, Dakar, 1966
- Southern Illinois University and area, 1964–present
- Case Western Reserve University, Cleveland, 1973
- International Institute of Ethnomusicology and Folklore,Caracas, Venezuela, 1974
- Artists-in-Residence/Lecturer Afro-Am Studies, University of California at Berkeley, 1976

Publications

Forewords
- Publications of Ruban Carambula, Uruguary and Earl Leaf, New York, 1949
- Black Dance in the United States, 1972
- Preface to Tropiques, magazine for French Colonies, 1952

Articles

- *Haiti,* Chicago Sun Times, July 1939
- *Les Pecheurs, Les Vierges,* Manuscripts, Chicago, 1939
- *La Boule Blanche,* Esquire, Sept. 1939, pseudonym Kaye Dunn
- *Thesis turned Broadway,* California Arts and Architecture, August 1941
- *The American Negro Dance and Its West Indian Affiliations,* Sterling Brown's Negro Caravan
- *Interrelation of Form and Function in Primitive Dance, Educational Dance,* October, 1941
- *Goombay,* Mademoiselle, November, 1945
- *Notes on the Dance,* Seven Arts, Doubleday, 1954
- *Notes on the Dance,* (reprint)
- *Ballet,* Argentina, Jan. 1955
- *Sketchbook of a Dancer in La Martinque,* Realities
- *Islands in Retrospect,* Show, 1963
- Field Technique for Tourists in the Caribbean, Travel, 1963

Short Stories

- *Audrey,* Phylon, Atlanta University review of Race and Culture
- *Afternoon into Night,* Bandwagon, Vol. XIII, London, June 1952, reprinted Langston Hughes Best Stories by Negro writers, 1967
- *Crime of Pablo Martinez,* Ellery Queen's Magazine, 1964

Books

- *Journey to Accompong,* Henry Holt, 1946
- *Journey to Accompong,* (reprint) Negro Universities Press, 1971
- *Las Danzas De Haiti,* Acta Anthropologica 114, Mexico November, 1947
- *Touch of Innocence,* Harcourt-Brace, September, 1959 & 69
- *Kasamance,* Third Press, New York, 1974
- *Island Possessed,* Doubleday 1969

Educational Activities

Research student of Social Anthropology, University of Chicago, Northwestern University, West Indies.

Fellowship, Rosenwald and Guggenheim Foundations

Supervisor, WPA Writer's Project, Chicago, subject: Drugs, Cults and Magic and Their Incidence Among Deprived People—The Black Muslims

Director and teacher of own schools of dance, theatre and cultural arts in Chicago, New York, Haiti, Stockholm, paris, and Italy. Twice Artist-in-Residence, Southern Illinois University, Carbondale and Edwardsville, Illinois

Educational Activities cont.: State Department United States Specialist Dakar, Senegal, 1966

Technical Cultural Advisor to the Presidency, Republic of Senegal, Dakar, Senegal, 1966

Consultant, International Institute of Ethnomusicology and Folklore, Caracas, Venezuela

Founder, Foundation for the Development and Preservation of Cultural Arts, Inc., not for profit, federally tax exempt, New York

Founder, Dunham Fund for Research and Development of Cultural Arts, Inc., Not for profit, federally tax exempt, East St. Louis, Illinois

Commencement speaker, MacMurray College, Jacksonville, IL, May 1972

Visiting Mather Scholar, Case Western Reserve University, Cleveland, Ohio, February, 1973

Visiting Professor, University of California at Berkeley, Berkeley, California, April–June 1976

Founder, Foundation Katherine Dunham, Pour la Promotion des Valeurs Noires, Port au Prince, Haiti

Founding Director, L'Institut de Recherche et de Conservation des Arts et de la Science du Vaudun (VIRCAS), Port au Prince, Haiti

Dance as a Cultural Art and its Role in Economic Development, lecturer and participant in the INternational Coloquium in Honor of the 70th Anniversary of President Leopold Sedar Senghor, Dakar, Senegal, October, 1976

Founding Director, Katherine Dunham Museum, East St. Louis, IL 1977

University Professor, Emerita Southern Illinois University, Edwardsville, IL, and Director of the Performing Arts Training Center of Southern Illinois University, East St. Louis, IL; Continuing research and writing

Awards

- Honorary Women's Scientific Fraternity, University of Chicago, 1937
- Chevalier, Haitian Legion of Honor and Merit, 1952
- Commander, Haitian Legion of Honor and Merit, 1952
- Grand Officer, Haitian Legion of Honor and Merit, 1968
- Honorary Citizen, Port au Prince, Haiti, 1957
- Laureate and Member, Lincoln Academy, State of Illinois, 1968
- Key to the City of East St. Louis, Illinois, 1968
- Professional Achievement Award, University of Chicago
- Alumni Association, University of Chicago, 1968
- Dance Pioneer Aware, Alvin Ailey American Dance Theatre, 1968
- Dance Magazine Aware, 1969
- Eight Lively Arts Award, 1969
- Improved Benevolent and Protective Order of Elks of the World Certificate of Merit, 1969
- Southern Illinois University Distinguished Service Aware, 1969
- St. Louis Argus Award, 1970,
- East St. Louis Monitor Award, 1970
- Katherine Dunham Day Award, Detroit, 1970
- Certificate of Merit, International Who's Who in Poetry, 1970 and 1971
- Dance Division Heritage Award AAHPER, Detroit, 1971
- East St. Louis Pro-Eight Award, 1970
- Woman for the Day, Radio Station WRTH, St. Louis, 1973
- Black Filmmakers Hall of Fame, 1974
- Grace Lee Stevens Civic and Charity Club Award, Chicago, 1974
- Female Artist Award, Hi-Phi-Hi Social Club, 1974

- Discovery Achievement Award, 1974
- American Dance Guild Award, St. Louis, 1975
- Outstanding Achievement Award, Black Alumni Club, University of California, Berkeley, California 1976
- Ten Year Merit Award, Southern Illinois University, Edwardsville, IL, 1977
- Cultural and Ethnic Affairs Award, Oakland Museum, Oakland, California, 1978
- Albert Schweeitzer Music Award, Carnegie Hall, New York, Jan., 1979
- Distinguished Achievement Award National Association of Negro Musicians, St. Louis, 1979
- Midwest Black Theatre Alliance Award, 1979
- Contribution to the Arts Award, Black Academy of Arts and Letters, 1972
- National Center of Afro-American Artists Award, Elma Lewis School of Fine Arts, Boston, 1972
- Black Merit Academy Award, 1972
- Black Heritage Commemorative Stamp—1st day cover of the Black Heritage covers "Legacies" series, honored under "Modern Dance" USPS Stamp, 1978
- Outstanding Accomplishments International Cultural Impressario" KMOX-TV/CBS, St. Louis, 1980
- Student Action for Education Award, Southern Illinois University, East St. Louis, 1980
- Distinguished Service Award, Institute for the Study of African Culture, St. Louis, 1980
- National Council for Black Studies Award Academic Excellence and Social Responsibility, Chicago, 1982
- Kennedy Center Honors Award, John F. Kennedy Center for the Performing Arts, Washington, D.C. December, 1983
- The Legion d'Honneur et Merite, Embassy of Haiti—Washington, D.C., December, 1983
- Plaque d'Honneur, Haitian—American Chamber of Commerce, Port-Au-Prince, Haiti, December, 1983.

Musical Compositions and Paintings

- Musical compositions and songs for stage and films
- Exhibitions of paintings in Paris, Milan, London, Sydney, Lima, Buenos Aires
- Member Italian Authors and Composers' Union, ASCAP

Recreation and Hobbies

Steambaths, Cooking, Writing and Painting

Memberships

- Advocates for the Arts, Charter Member
- Black Filmmakers Hall of Fame, Inductee & Board Member
- Black Academy of Arts and Letters (BAAL), Awardee and Member
- Dance Scope, Consulting Editor
- Dunham Fund for Research and Development of Cultural Arts, Inc., President
- Foundation for the Study of Arts and Sciences of the Vodun, Founder
- Foundations for the Development and Preservation of Cultural Arts, Inc., Vice President
- Institute of the Black World, Board Member
- Interamerican Institute for Ethnomusicology and Folklore, (IN-IDEF) Caracas, Venezuela, Consultant
- Chairman's National Commission to Expand the Scope Constituency of Black Participation at the John F. Kennedy Center for Performing Arts, Washington, D.C., Board Member
- Organization of American States, Consultant
- National Advisory Council on Aging, Board Member
- Performing Arts Panel for the Aging, Member
- Review Committee National Endowment for the Humanities, Consultant
- Fullbright Fellow, State Department International Education, Fellow

Published Books By Or About Katherine Dunham

By Katherine Dunham

Journey to Accompong, by Katherine Dunham, Henry Holt & Co., Inc., New York, 1946.

Las Danzas De Haiti, by Katherine Dunham, Acta Anthropologica, 11:4 Mexico, November 1947. (In Spanish and English)

Les Dances De Haiti, by Katherine Dunham, Paris: Fasquel Press, 1957.

A Touch of Innocence, by Katherine Dunham, Harbrace Paperbound Library, Harcourt, Brace & World, Inc., New York, 1959 and 1969.

Island Possessed, by Katherine Dunham, Doubleday and Co., Inc., Garden City, New York, 1969.

Journey to Accompong, by Katherine Dunham, Negro Universities Press, Division of Greenwood Press, Inc., Westport, Connecticut, Reprinted in 1971.

Kasamance, by Katherine Dunham, Third Press, Joseph Okpaku Publishing Co., New York, 1974.

Dances of Haiti, by Katherine Dunham, Center for Afro-American Studies, UCLA, Los Angeles, California, 1983.

About Katherine Dunham

Katherine Dunham, Her dancers, Singers, Musicians, (Text in English and in French), Edited and with an Introduction by Richard Buckle, Ballet Publications Ltd., William Clowes & Sons, Ltd., London & Beccles, 1948.

Dance: The Story of Katherine Dunham, by Ruth Biemiller, A Doubleday Signal Book, Doubleday & Co., Inc., Garden City, New York, 1969.

African Rhythm, American Dance, by Terry Harnan, A Borzoi Book, Alfred A. Knopf, Inc., New York, 1974.

KAISO! Katherine Dunham, An Anthology of Writings, Edited by VeVe Clark and Margaret B. Wilkerson, Institute for the Study of Social Change, CCEW Women's Center, University of California, Berkeley, 1978.

Katherine Dunham, A Biography, by Ruth Beckford, Marcel Dekker, Inc., New York, 1979.

Katherine Dunham, by James Haskins, Coward, McCann & Geoghegan, Inc., New York, 1982.

Katherine Dunham: Reflections on the Social and Political Contexts of Afro-American Dance, by Dr. Joyce Aschenbrenner, CORD Publishing Co., 1980.

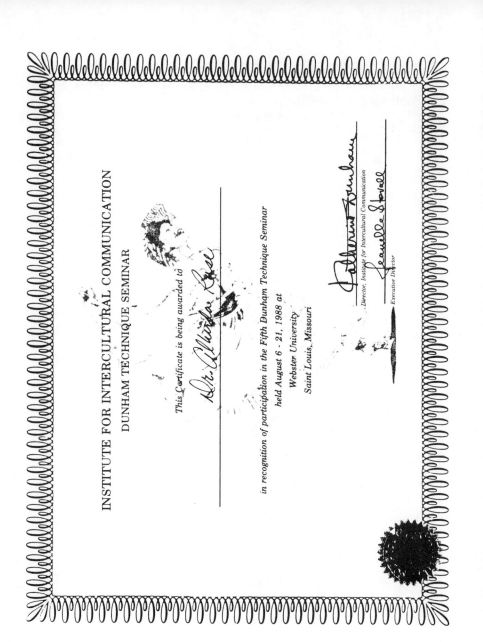

INSTITUTE FOR INTERCULTURAL COMMUNICATION

DUNHAM TECHNIQUE SEMINAR

This Certificate is being awarded to

Dr. Albirtha Bru

in recognition of participation in the Fifth Dunham Technique Seminar

held August 6 - 21, 1988 at

Webster University

Saint Louis, Missouri

Director, Institute for Intercultural Communication

Executive Director

The Katherine Dunham School of Arts and Research

including

DUNHAM SCHOOL OF DANCE AND THEATRE
DEPARTMENT OF CULTURAL STUDIES – INSTITUTE FOR CARIBBEAN RESEARCH
LA BOULE BLANCHE

THIS IS TO CERTIFY THAT

JANE DOE

has satisfactorily completed the necessary requirements for

MASTER TEACHER

course of study prescribed by this school and
having met the requirements is entitled to this

CERTIFICATE

given at , this 2nd day

of November 1989

DIRECTOR

CERTIFICATE OF CREDITS

for qualification as

INSTRUCTOR *ARTIST* *FIELD RESEARCH WORKER* *MASTER*

in the schools of

DANCE	DRAMA	CULTURAL STUDIES
PRIMITIVE RHYTHMS	ELEMENTARY ACTING	FUNDAMENTAL ANTHROPOLOGY
DUNHAM TECHNIQUE I	ACTING TECHNIQUES	INTRODUCTORY PSYCHOLOGY
DUNHAM TECHNIQUE II	BODY MOVEMENT FOR ACTORS	INTRODUCTORY PHILOSOPHY AND AESTHETICS
CLASSICAL BALLET	TECHNIQUES OF PANTOMIME	
MODERN DANCE FORMS	VOICE AND SPEECH	CONVERSATIONAL FRENCH
RHYTHM-TAP	HISTORY OF DRAMA	FRENCH CREOLE
CLASSIC SPANISH TECHNIQUE	CLASSIC DRAMA	SPANISH
		AFRO-CUBAN
PERCUSSION	PLAYWRITING	RUSSIAN
		BRAZILIAN
EUKINETICS	SCENE DEVELOPMENT	
CHOREUTICS	RADIO THEORY AND PRACTICE	DANCE FILM HISTORICAL AND CURRENT
DANCE NOTATION	STAGE MANAGEMENT AND DIRECTION	MUSIC APPRECIATION
CARIBBEAN AND SOUTH AMERICAN SOCIAL DANCES	VISUAL DESIGN	SURVEY OF HISTORICAL MOVEMENT
	COSTUME EXECUTION	
DANCE HISTORY	MAKE-UP FOR STAGE AND CAMERA	FORM AND FUNCTION
FORM AND SPACE		GUIDED READING

DUNHAM TECHNIQUE SEMINAR

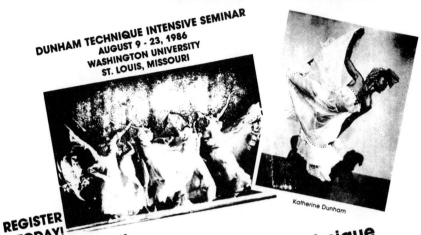

DUNHAM TECHNIQUE INTENSIVE SEMINAR
AUGUST 9 - 23, 1986
WASHINGTON UNIVERSITY
ST. LOUIS, MISSOURI

Katherine Dunham

REGISTER TODAY!

- Individual Sessions $10.00
- Daily Sessions $45.00
- 78 Intensive Sessions $350.00

Learn Dunham Technique from Master Dancers

★ Primitive Rhythms
★ Seminars, Technique, Anthropology
★ Films on Choreography and Dunham Company, and Philosophy

CUT OUT ✂ — — — — —

DUNHAM TECHNIQUE SEMINAR
AUGUST 9 - 23, 1986

NAME: _____

ADDRESS: _____

CITY/STATE/ZIP: _____

TELEPHONE:(DAY) _____

(NIGHT) _____

All fees tax-deductible. Master Card/Visa accepted.
Make checks/money orders payable to: Dunham Technique Seminar
532 North 10th Street
East St. Louis, IL 62201

Level of Dance Experience: _____ Beginner
(Check one)
_____ Intermediate
_____ Advanced

Will you want course credit (only
thru San Francisco State University)? _____ YES
_____ NO

For more information, contact:

Dr. Alberda Rose   Gezelle Glass
618/271-3367   314/361-1991